Body
fitness
AND EXERCISE

Body fitness

AND EXERCISE

*Basic theory
and practice
for therapists*

MO ROSSER

Hodder & Stoughton

A MEMBER OF THE HODDER HEADLINE GROUP

British Library Cataloguing in Publication Data

Benton, Peter
  Inside Stories. – Book 2
  I. Title   II. Benton, Susan
  823.0108

ISBN 0-340-50359-9

First published 1993
Impression number   10 9 8 7 6 5 4
Year   2003 2002 2001 2000

Typeset by Keyset Composition, Colchester, Essex
Printed in Great Britain for Hodder & Stoughton Educational, a division
of Hodder Headline Plc, 338 Euston Road, London NW1 3BH
by J W Arrowsmith Ltd, Bristol.

Contents

Ef Côf am rhieni annwyl
William Aldwyn a Catherine Read

Acknowledgements

I am indebted to many people for their advice and support during the preparation of this book. In particular, my thanks to Sue Wandless of the London College of Fashion for reading and advising on the text. For their encouragement and patience, I thank Elsie Rosser, Sue Rosser and Helen Price, and my husband, Gwyn, for his consistent support. Special thanks also to Suzie Robertson and Jeff Rosser, who meticulously typed, prepared and organised the manuscript.

The author and publisher would like to thank the following, for permission and assistance in the reproduction of copyright photographs and material: Accoson Ltd, fig. 10.5; British Medical Association, fig. 10.4; Pharma-Plast Ltd, fig. 8.2; Powersport International Ltd, fig. 8.5 & p. 91; Ragdale Hall Health Hydro, fig. 10.1 & p. 135; Vitalograph Ltd, fig. 10.3. Permission has been granted by the publisher, Edward Arnold, for the reproduction of several figures from: Sears, W. Gordon (1985) *Anatomy and Physiology for Nurses*, eds. R. S. Winwood and E. Sears, London: Edward Arnold (figs. 2.8, 3.4–3.17, 3.19, 3.21, 4.6, 5.1, 5.2, 5.4).

Every effort has been made to obtain permission for the reproduction of copyright material. Any queries regarding such should be addressed to the publisher.

PART A *Principles relating to exercise*

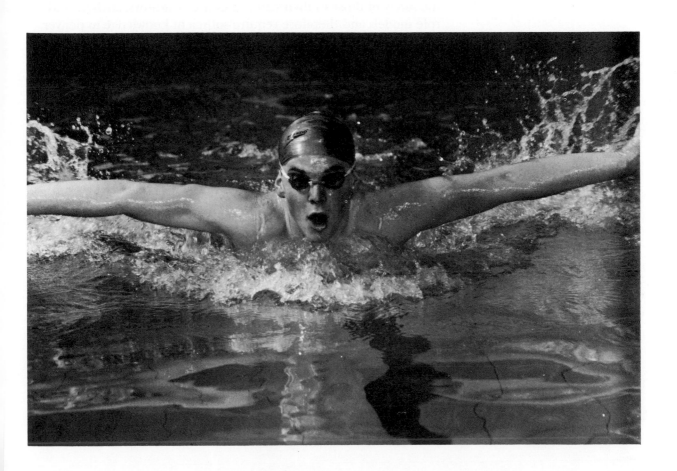

Introduction

There has been an enormous growth in the fitness industry over the past few years as people have become aware of the beneficial effects of exercise. Regular exercise improves fitness, is beneficial to health and will reduce the risk of developing many diseases. It creates a sense of well-being and produces greater energy.

Teachers of exercise have to be aware of their responsibility for the safety of those in their care. They are educators, advisers and role models and therefore require sufficient knowledge to deliver safe and effective exercise and to give accurate advice. Beneficial effects are only derived from exercise that is appropriate and correctly performed. Inappropriate exercise casually performed will result in trauma, injury, pain and stiffness.

This books covers the basic theory of fitness and exercise and will enable the student to construct suitable programmes to meet a variety of needs. It is impossible to cover all types of exercise in one book and further reading about specific training regimes is required. Students must keep abreast of new developments and use knowledge carefully for the benefit of their clients.

CHAPTER 1

The benefits of exercise

Research has shown that regular exercise is beneficial for all age groups. In response to exercise the body makes certain physiological changes. The extent of these changes will depend on the type of exercise and on the body systems that are subjected to stress. Appropriate exercises regularly practised will improve physical fitness, promote health and reduce the risk of developing many diseases. The beneficial effects derived from exercise are both physiological and psychological.

The physiological benefits are:

- improvement in cardio-vascular function, i.e. heart and circulation;
- improvement in respiratory function, i.e. lungs and breathing;
- improvement in muscle tone, strength and stamina, which in turn improves posture and body contours (shape);
- improvement in the flexibility and tensile strength of tendons and ligaments. This will increase the range of movement at joints and reduce the likelihood of trauma;
- improvement in the condition of joints. Exercise increases the production of synovial fluid, which lubricates and nourishes the cartilage;
- improvement in bone density, which will combat osteoporosis;
- improvement in neuro-muscular co-ordination, which improves skills such as rhythm, balance, timing, reaction time and co-ordination;
- increase in metabolic rate, with reduction in fat reserves. Muscle tissue has a high metabolic rate, therefore the more muscle tissue on the body, the higher the metabolic rate. This will increase demand for fuel and thus reduce fat stores;
- lowering of blood cholesterol levels;
- reduction in trauma and pain due to improved posture, strength and flexibility;

- reduction in the risk of developing debilitating diseases such as hypertension (high blood pressure), heart disease, types of diabetes. Exercise reduces stress, which is a contributory factor in many of these illnesses.

The psychological benefits are:

- feelings of well-being, achievement and euphoria;
- an increase in self-confidence and self-esteem;
- reduction in stress levels;
- promotion of relaxation and sleep.

To achieve these benefits, exercises must be carefully selected and accurately and carefully performed. Exercise should always be specific to the individual, and the degree of ease or difficulty should be appropriate for the level of fitness. Inappropriate exercises that are too difficult or are casually and excessively performed can result in damage and pain.

DAMAGING EFFECTS OF INAPPROPRIATE EXERCISE

- muscle strain, tears and soreness;
- ligamentous sprains, overstretching and tears;
- joint stresses;
- bone stresses;
- inflammation of tendons, bursae and joint capsules, namely tendonitis, bursitis and capsulitis;
- pain, which adversely affects daily activities, relaxation and sleep. Pain may also produce feelings of tension, stress, depression, disappointment and low self-esteem.

The effect on the cardio-vascular system – heart, blood and vessels

During exercise, contracting muscles require a steady supply of oxygen for energy production, over and above that required for normal activities. Regular aerobic exercise will improve cardio-vascular fitness. Aerobic exercise involves repetitive movements of large muscle groups and includes activities such as walking, jogging, swimming and cycling. The heart must respond to meet the demand for oxygen and nutrients and to prevent the build-up of waste products.

The heart and vessels respond and adapt in the following ways:

- The heart increases in size and volume;

- The heart pumps out more blood with each beat (stroke volume) and therefore pumps out more blood per minute (cardiac output);
- Because the heart pumps out more blood with each beat, fewer beats per minute are necessary and the heart rate decreases. A normal heart rate is around 72–76 beats per minute, but endurance athletes such as marathon runners may have heart rates as low as 40 beats per minute. This reduces the work load of the heart;
- There is an increase in the density of the capillary networks supplying blood to cardiac and skeletal muscles;
- The blood vessels increase in size and number and blood flow is increased. This improves the delivery of oxygen and nutrients and the removal of waste products;
- Increased levels of haemoglobin increase the oxygen-carrying capacity of the blood.

Regular aerobic activities, therefore, greatly improve the function and endurance of the heart. Carefully graded and controlled exercises form part of cardiac rehabilitation programmes following heart problems and heart attacks.

The effect on the respiratory system – the respiratory tract and lungs

- The demand for more oxygen and the increase in the production of carbon dioxide increases the rate and depth of ventilation. During exercise the volume of air breathed in and out of the lungs may be 30 times greater than that breathed at rest.
- The elasticity and condition of the lung tissue improves.
- The blood supply to and from the lungs increases.
- The condition of the muscles that move the thorax – the intercostals and diaphragm – improves as they are made to work harder.

EXERCISE AND ASTHMA

Asthma sufferers may exercise with caution, but must not over-exert. One must always bear in mind that physical exertion can sometimes trigger an asthmatic attack. This is referred to as exercise-induced asthma. If breathing difficulties are experienced for longer than normal, i.e. over five minutes, and there is obvious distress, then medical advice should be sought quickly. Asthmatics should always have bronchodilators to hand, and must learn to recognise distress signals and take appropriate steps to control the condition. However, research has shown that increased aerobic fitness can reduce the frequency of attacks. Asthmatics derive benefit from exercise performed in short bursts with frequent rest intervals. It is better to exercise indoors than outdoors, in order to avoid cold air, pollen and other allergens. Indoor swimming is ideal as it provides gentle exercise in a warm, humid atmosphere.

The effect on skeletal muscle

Muscle tissue responds in several ways to training and overload:

- Strength and bulk will improve in response to resistance exercises;
- Flexibility will improve with stretch exercises;
- Endurance will improve in response to repetitive exercises.

STRENGTH AND BULK

- Muscle strength will increase, providing the muscle is made to work against sub-maximal or maximal loads. As the muscle strengthens the load must be progressively increased.
- More motor units are recruited, which increases the strength of contraction.
- Muscle size (bulk) increases. Research to date suggests that this is due to an increase in the size and number of myofibrils, rather than to an increase in muscle fibres, but this is still in dispute. The increase in bulk is largely due to the increase in the contractile proteins myosin and actin. Generally, males will bulk more readily than females. This is due to higher levels of the male hormone testosterone, which is necessary for the synthesis of actin and myosin. Females show little bulking, but will develop strength by progressive weight training. Some muscles bulk more readily than others, for example the biceps and quadriceps bulk readily, while the abdominals do not.
- There is an increase in stored energy supplies (ATP, PC) and enzymes, giving a greater source of quick energy.

ENDURANCE

Muscle endurance improves when a muscle is made to contract repeatedly against low or moderate resistance. As a result of endurance training other changes occur:

- an increase in the number and size of blood vessels supplying blood to muscle fibres;

- an increase in the density of the capillary networks supplying blood to muscle fibres;
- an increase in the blood flow, thus improving the delivery of oxygen and the removal of waste;
- an increase in the number of mitochondria in the muscle cells, and therefore greater efficiency in utilising oxygen;
- an increase in glycogen stores. The increased availability of oxygen and glycogen raises the anaerobic threshold, so that the muscles use aerobic energy for longer periods, thus reducing levels of lactic acid. The muscles can continue contracting for longer periods without fatigue.

FLEXIBILITY

Flexibility exercises gently stretch musculo-tendinous components at a joint. Flexibility exercises at the end of an exercise programme will reduce muscle soreness.

The effect at the joints

- Movement at the joints stimulates the secretion of synovial fluid. This lubricates and nourishes the cartilage, improving its condition and allowing smoother movements at the joints.
- Stretching or flexibility exercises will maintain and increase the range of movements at the joints. Joint range may be increased actively or passively. An active stretch is a free movement performed by the client (see chapter 8). A passive stretch is performed by the therapist or partner applying pressure at the end of the range while the client's muscles are relaxed. This must be performed with great care and must only be undertaken after thorough training.

The effect on connective tissue structures

The flexibility of connective tissue structures around the joints, i.e. the supporting ligaments, tendons and capsule, will improve with regular exercise. This increased suppleness will reduce the likelihood of injuries such as sprains, tears and ruptures. The loss of flexibility due to ageing or immobilisation responds well to regular exercise undertaken to restore and maintain function, but every precaution must be taken not to produce excessive stress or strain.

The effect on the bones

Bones are strengthened in response to the stresses imposed upon them, particularly through exercise. More calcium salts are deposited and the condition and strength of the bones improve. Exercise is particularly beneficial for post-menopausal women, as it can delay and protect against the development of osteoporosis. (This is a condition where the bones become brittle and fracture easily due to a lack of mineral salts.)

The effect on the metabolism

Exercise increases the metabolic rate (the rate at which the body uses energy). The metabolic rate of skeletal muscle can vary to a greater degree than that of any other tissue. An exercising muscle has a metabolic rate up to 50 times higher than a muscle at rest. It therefore expends 50 times more energy. Glycogen is the first source of energy, but when these stores are depleted during prolonged exercise, energy is obtained from fat (fatty acids and glycerol). This is taken from body stores, with resultant weight loss. It is an advantage to have a high proportion of muscle tissue, as its high metabolic rate utilises more energy than other tissues. Exercises increase muscle bulk, which in turn increases energy consumption. By exercising regularly low energy consumers become high energy consumers. Thus a regular aerobic programme and a low-calorie diet will result in a reduction of body fat and also in lower blood cholesterol levels.

It is important to remember that the fat will be taken from fat stores all over the body. It is not possible to 'spot reduce', in other words to take fat from an area such as the hips by exercising the muscles of the hip region, or from the abdomen by doing curl-ups. These exercises expend little energy and it is unlikely that fat will be utilised as an energy source. Prolonged steady-state aerobic programmes are the most effective way of losing weight, particularly if accompanied by a low-fat and low-sugar diet.

The effect on neuro-muscular co-ordination

The nervous system controls muscle contraction and the resulting movements. The brain co-ordinates the patterns of movement that result in skilled performance. Regular practice and repetition reinforce these patterns and improve co-ordination, speed and skill.

CHAPTER 2

Anatomy and physiology

To appreciate fully the effects of exercise and to educate their clients, all exercise therapists must have a sound basic knowledge of anatomy and physiology. Anatomy is the study of the structure of the body. Physiology is the study of the functions of the body.

An in-depth study of these subjects is not within the scope of this book and the therapist should refer to a specialist anatomy and physiology textbook. This first section will review the body systems and elaborate specifically on those involved in movement, namely the skeletal and muscular systems.

The organisational levels of the body

Chemical → Cellular → Tissue → Organ → Body System

CHEMICAL

Beginning at the very basic level, we have the chemicals that are essential for maintaining life. Reactions in which these chemicals are combined or broken down underlie all the processes necessary for sustaining life.

CELLULAR

The cells are the basic structural and functional units of the body. All the activities that maintain life are carried out by the cells. The body is made up of billions of cells: they all have a similar basic structure, but change slightly to suit their function, for example blood cells differ from fat cells.

THE STRUCTURE OF A TYPICAL CELL

THE CELL MEMBRANE OR PLASMA MEMBRANE

This is the outer layer or boundary of the cell. It gives shape to the cell and protects it, separating things inside the cell (intracellular) from those outside the cell (extracellular). It regulates the passage of substances in and out of the cell.

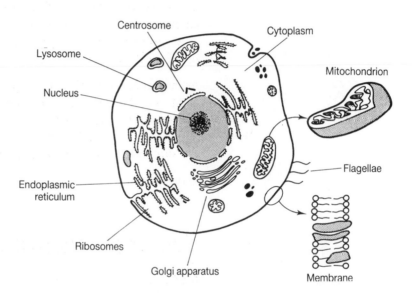

Figure 2.1 *A typical cell*

THE CYTOPLASM

This is a soft, jelly-like substance where the functions of the cell are carried out. It contains various structures called organelles (mini-organs), each of which has a specific function. Also in the cytoplasm are various chemical substances called inclusions.

THE ORGANELLES

These mini-organs each have a characteristic shape and a specific role to perform. The type and number of organelles in different kinds of cells vary depending on the activities of the cell; for example, muscle cells have large numbers of mitochondria, because they have a high level of energy output.

- The largest of the organelles is the nucleus. It controls the activities of the cell and it contains the body's genetic material (DNA).

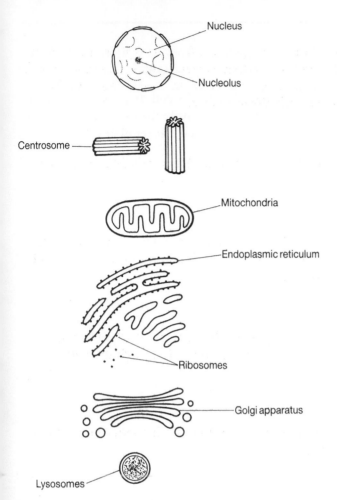

Figure 2.2 *Organelles found in the cell*

Other organelles include:

- Mitochondria, which generate energy;
- Ribosomes, which synthesise protein;
- Lysosomes, which digest and deal with waste;
- The Golgi apparatus is concerned with the production of membrane and protein lipids and glycoproteins;
- Endoplasmic reticulum – a series of channels for transporting substances within the cell;
- The centrosome, involved in cell division.

THE INCLUSIONS

These are chemical substances produced by cells. They may not be present in all cells. For example, melanin is a pigment found in certain cells of the skin and hair; it protects the body by screening out ultra-violet light, and gives the skin its brown colour on exposure to sunlight. Glycogen is found in liver and skeletal muscle cells, and provides quick energy. Lipids are found in fat cells and are broken down to provide energy when required.

THE CHARACTERISTICS OF CELLS

All living things, whether they be single-celled or multi-celled organisms, have certain characteristics or functions in common that are essential to life:

METABOLISM

This is the sum total of all the cells' chemical activities. There are two phases of metabolism:

- *Catabolism* is the breaking down of chemical substances derived from food to provide the energy and heat needed to sustain life;
- *Anabolism* uses the energy of catabolism to build new chemical compounds and repair tissues.

RESPIRATION

Cells are capable of producing energy from food substances taken in by or stored in the body. When oxygen is utilised in this process, it is termed *aerobic respiration*; when oxygen is not utilised in the process, it is termed *anaerobic respiration.*

GROWTH

Cells grow in size up to a certain limit. When this limit is reached the cells divide.

REPRODUCTION

When the growth of cells is complete, they divide to produce two daughter cells that are identical to each other. This process of cell division is known as *mitosis.*

EXCRETION

Cells are capable of getting rid of the waste products resulting from metabolism; these pass out of the cell through the cell membrane.

IRRITABILITY

Cells are capable of responding to stimuli, which may be physical, chemical or thermal.

MOVEMENT

Some cells are capable of movement. They move by pushing out fingers of cytoplasm called pseudopodia or by the movement of flagellae.

TISSUES

The tissues of the body are made up of groups of similar cells that work together to perform a specific function. All the cells of one tissue will be the same, but the cells of different tissues will be modified to suit the function of that particular tissue. There are four main types of tissue in the body:

- *Epithelial tissue* covers the body's surfaces, lines the organs and tubes and forms glands;
- *Connective tissue* supports and protects organs, binds and connects tissues and organs together and provides storage of fat for energy reserves;
- *Muscular tissue* is able to contract and relax to produce movement;

- *Nervous tissue* initiates and transmits impulses to co-ordinate the activities of the body. It is the communication system of the body.

EPITHELIAL TISSUE OR EPITHELIUM

This tissue covers external body surfaces and forms the outer covering of body organs. It also forms the inner lining of organs, tracts, vessels and ducts. Glandular epithelium lines glands and secretes substances.

Epithelium is composed of closely-packed cells. There are two main classifications:

- simple epithelium, which is a single layer of cells;
- stratified or compound epithelium, which consists of many layers of cells.

It may be further sub-classified according to the shape of the cells. The many types of epithelium may be summarised as shown in Tables 2.1 and 2.2.

Glandular epithelium contains cells that secrete substances and is found in glands. Exocrine glands secrete substances into ducts or directly onto surfaces: for example, sweat glands secrete sweat, salivary glands secrete saliva and various digestive tract glands secrete digestive juices. Endocrine glands, for example the adrenal and thyroid glands, secrete hormones directly into the blood. These chemicals regulate certain physiological processes.

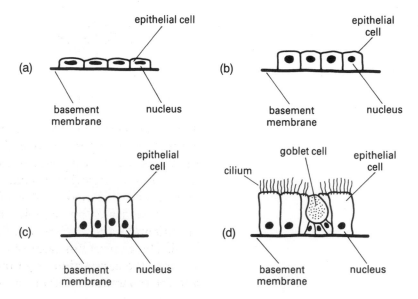

Figure 2.3 *Simple epithelium*

Table 2.1 *Types of simple epithelium*

Name	Type	Location
Squamous	flat cells	lines heart and blood vessels, alveoli
Cuboidal	cube-shaped cells	lines kidney tubules, ducts of glands
Columnar	cells like columns	lines stomach and digestive tract
Columnar ciliated	columns with hair-like cilia	lines respiratory tract and fallopian tubes

Table 2.2 *Types of compound epithelium*

Name	Type	Location
Squamous	layers of flat cells	non-keratinised: lines mouth, tongue, oesophagus
		keratinised: forms outer layer of skin
Cuboidal	layers of flat cube-shaped cells	ducts of sweat glands
Columnar	layers of columnar cells	lines parts of male urethra, anus
Transitional	layers of cells which compress and allow tissues to be distended	lines bladder, ureters and urethra

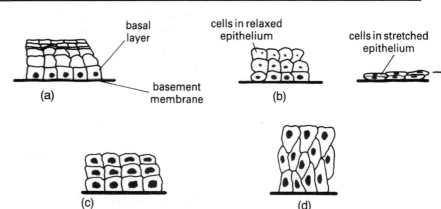

Figure 2.4 *Compound epithelium*

CONNECTIVE TISSUE

This is the most widely distributed tissue in the body. There are many different types of connective tissue, all with specific functions. Connective tissue is composed of a ground substance or matrix in which are found widely scattered cells and fibres. The type of matrix or intercellular substance determines the type of connective tissue; for example, some types of tissue are fluid, some are soft and some are firm and flexible, while others are hard and rigid. The general functions of connective tissue are protection, support, the connection or joining together of various structures and the separation of others, and the storage of energy reserves.

Table 2.3 *Types of connective tissue*

Name	Structure	Location/function
Areolar tissue	loose moist tissue with a viscous matrix and a loose, irregular arrangement of fibres: white fibres for strength and yellow fibres for elasticity. A variety of cells are found scattered throughout	widely distributed as dermis of skin and under the skin as superficial fascia; between other tissues and around organs. It gives strength, elasticity and support
Adipose tissue	loose connective tissue, with large numbers of specialised cells, called *adipocytes*, for fat storage. The cytoplasm and nucleus of the cell are pushed to one side and fat fills the cell	subcutaneous layer of skin, the amount varying between thin and obese people; around heart and kidney; in the marrow of long bones; as padding around joints. Regular aerobic exercise will utilise the fats from these stores as a source of energy
Dense or white fibrous connective tissue	composed of closely-packed bundles of fibres, mainly white collagen fibres, interspersed with cells	forms tendons and aponeuroses that attach muscle to bone, and ligaments that hold bones together; provides a protective covering for organs, e.g. kidney, heart, liver, testes
Yellow elastic tissue	composed mainly of yellow elastic fibres with few fibroblasts. This tissue gives elasticity and strength, recoiling to its original shape after stretching	forms the walls of arteries, trachea, bronchial tubes and the lungs. It allows organs to stretch and recoil
Reticular tissue	reticular fibres form a delicate network with cells wrapped around them	forms delicate support within organs such as spleen, lymph nodes, liver
Cartilage (three types)		
hyaline cartilage	consists of a gelatinous intercellular matrix with fine collagen fibres and cells called *chondrocytes*. Hyaline cartilage is smooth, tough, resilient and flexible. It is milky white with a bluish tinge. It is commonly called gristle	covers the ends or articulating surfaces of bones; forms the costal cartilages, the rings of the trachea and bronchi and the nasal septum; provides a smooth surface to minimise friction at joints. With age, injury or disease this cartilage may be damaged or eroded, and friction at the joint increases as bone rubs on bone, producing pain and stiffness
fibro-cartilage	similar to hyaline, but the matrix contains bundles of collagen fibres with widely dispersed chondrocytes. The fibres give strength, toughness and flexibility. It gives a slight cushioning effect when compressed	found in the symphysis pubis, inter-vertebral discs and the menisci of the knee. It supports and cushions. Severe compression and abnormal movements can damage discs and menisci. These are common injuries in sport and exercise (see chapter 15)

elastic cartilage	similar to hyaline, but the matrix consists of freely branching elastic fibres with dispersed chondrocytes. It is flexible and resilient. It gives support and shape	found in the epiglottis and external ear, giving shape and support
Bone or osseous tissue (two types)		
Compact bone	hard, dense, ivory-like tissue	forms the outer layer of bones
Cancellous bone	sponge-like structure with trabeculae and large spaces	found inside most bones
Blood	fluid connective tissue consisting of plasma and circulating cells	transports substances around the body. Regulates body healing. Prevents blood loss by coagulation

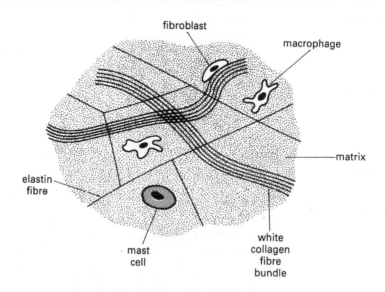

Figure 2.5 *Areolar tissue*

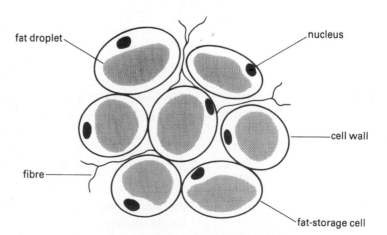

Figure 2.6 *Adipose tissue*

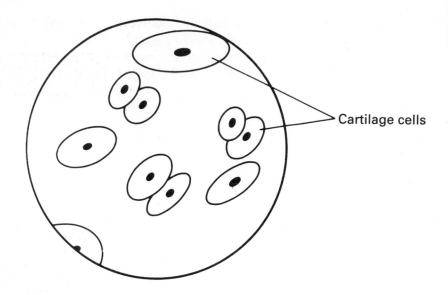

Figure 2.7 *Hyaline cartilage*

MUSCLE TISSUE

Muscle tissue is highly specialised, in that it is capable of contraction and relaxation. There are three types of muscle tissue:

- *Skeletal muscle* (voluntary; striated) is attached to bones. When skeletal muscle contracts it pulls on the bones and produces movement. It also maintains posture and produces body heat. The cells of skeletal muscles are long cylindrical fibres with many nuclei (multi-nucleated); they have a striped or 'striated' appearance. These muscle fibres are arranged in bundles and many bundles group together to form a muscle. See chapter 5 for further detail.

- *Cardiac muscle* (involuntary; striated) forms the wall of the heart. When cardiac muscle contracts it pumps blood around the body. The cells or fibres of cardiac muscles are quadrilateral in shape and contain only one nucleus. The cells branch, forming a network. The cells are separated from each other by thickened discs called intercalated discs.

- *Smooth muscle* (involuntary; non-striated) is found in the walls of blood vessels, the stomach, the intestine, the gall bladder and the urinary bladder. This muscle contracts to constrict blood vessels or to move food through the digestive tract and eliminate waste. The cells are spindle-shaped and contain a single nucleus.

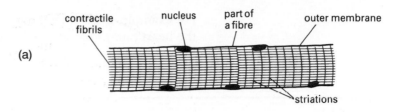

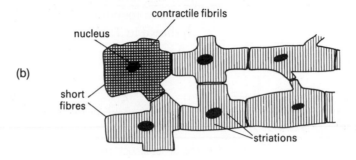

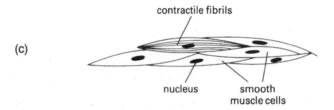

Figure 2.8 *Types of muscle tissue*

NERVOUS TISSUE

This tissue forms the nervous system. It consists of two types of cells: *neurones* and *neuroglia.*

Neurones pick up stimuli and conduct impulses to other neurones, to muscle fibres or to glands. There are three types:

- *Motor neurones* conduct impulses from the brain and spinal cord to muscles and glands.
- *Sensory neurones* conduct impulses from the sensory organs to the brain and spinal cord.
- *Interneurones* conduct impulses from one neurone to another.

Neuroglia support and protect neurones.

ORGANS

Many tissues join together to form the organs of the body. Each organ has a specific function or functions to perform.

For example, the stomach digests food, the lungs exchange gases, the heart pumps blood, the kidneys filter fluids and form urine, the ovaries produce and release ova. Organs combine to make up the systems of the body.

BODY SYSTEM

Each body system consists of many organs that co-operate to perform various functions. All the systems are interrelated and function together to maintain life. There are eleven body systems, as shown in Table 2.4.

Table 2.4 *The eleven body systems*

System	Location	Function
Integumentary system	the skin and all its structures; nails; hair; sweat and sebaceous (oil) glands	protects; regulates temperature; eliminates waste; makes vitamin D; receives stimuli
Skeletal system	the bones, joints and cartilages	supports; protects; aids movement; stores minerals; protects cells that produce blood cells
Muscular system	usually refers to skeletal muscle, but includes cardiac and smooth muscle	produces movement; maintains posture; produces heat
Nervous system	brain; spinal cord; nerves; sense organs	communicates and co-ordinates body functions
Cardio-vascular system	heart; blood vessels; blood	transports substances around the body; helps regulate body temperature; prevents blood loss by blood clotting
Lymphatic system	lymphatic vessels, nodes, lymph ducts; spleen; tonsils; thymus gland	returns proteins and plasma to blood; carries fat from intestine to blood; filters body fluid, forms white blood cells, protects against disease
Respiratory system	pharynx, larynx, trachea, bronchi and lungs	supplies oxygen and removes carbon dioxide
Digestive system	gastro-intestinal tract, i.e. mouth, pharynx, oesophagus, stomach, small intestine, large intestine, rectum, anus; salivary glands; gall bladder, liver and pancreas	physical and chemical breakdown of food; absorption of nutrients and elimination of waste
Urinary system	kidneys, ureters, bladder and urethra	helps to regulate chemical composition of blood; helps to balance the acid/alkali content of the body; eliminates urine

| Reproductive system | Female: breasts, ovaries, uterus, uterine tubes, vagina, external genitalia
Male: testes, epididymides, vas deferens, spermatic cords, seminal vesicles, ejaculatory ducts, prostate gland, penis | involved in reproduction and the production of sex hormones |
| Endocrine system | consists of ductless glands which produce and secrete hormones directly into the blood | hormones regulate a wide variety of body activities such as nutrition and growth, and they help maintain homeostasis |

QUESTIONS

1 List the organisational levels of the body.
2 Give three functions of the cell membrane.
3 Name the organelles that carry out the following functions:
   a synthesise protein
   b deal with waste
   c generate energy.
4 Define the term *metabolism*, and name the two phases involved.
5 Complete the following sentences:
   .... group together to form body tissues. Body systems are made up of many ....
6 List all the types of epithelial tissue and give the location of each.

7 a Name the tissue that stores body fat.
   b List three locations where fat is stored.
8 a List the three types of cartilage.
   b Name the cartilage that covers the articulating surfaces of bones.
9 Give the location of the following muscle tissues:
   a skeletal
   b smooth
   c cardiac.
   Draw a simple diagram of each tissue.
10 Name and give the function of the three types of neurone.

CHAPTER 3

The bones of the skeletal system

The anatomical position

Before we can describe body movement, we must have a basic position or static posture that is used as a common reference point for describing surfaces, relationships and directions of movement. This is known as the anatomical position.

In the anatomical position the body is upright, with feet slightly apart and toes pointing forward. The arms hang at the sides with the palms of the hands facing forwards. (Note the difference from the normal standing position, where the palms of the hands face the sides of the body.)

With the body in this position the directions of joint movements can be described in terms of planes and axes of movement.

BODY PLANES

These are imaginary surfaces along which movements take place. There are three planes: they lie at right angles to each other:

- The *Sagittal Plane* lies parallel to the sagittal suture of the skull. This plane divides the body into right and left parts. The Median Sagittal divides the body into equal right and left parts;
- The *Coronal or Frontal Plane* lies parallel to the coronal suture of the skull. This plane divides the body into front and back;
- The *Horizontal or Transverse Plane* is parallel to a flat floor. This plane divides the body into upper and lower parts.

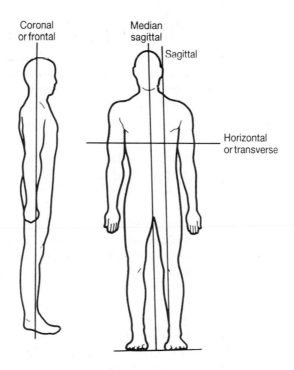

Figure 3.1 *Body planes*

AXES

The axis of a movement is a line around which the movement takes place (in the same way as a top spins about its axis). It is always at right angles to the plane of movement.

There are three axes of movement:

- *sagittal* – from back to front parallel to the sagittal suture of the skull;
- *coronal/frontal* – from side to side parallel to the coronal suture of the skull;
- *vertical* – straight up and down (vertical to the floor).

Examples of the planes and axes of certain movements when the body is in the anatomical position:

- flexion (bending) of the elbow is movement in a sagittal plane with a frontal axis;
- abduction of the hip (taking it out to the side) is movement in a frontal plane with a sagittal axis;
- turning the head from right to left is movement in a horizontal plane with a vertical axis.

TERMINOLOGY

It is important to be familiar with the terms used to describe surfaces of the body in the anatomical position and the position of structures relative to each other. These are shown in Figure 3.2 and described in Table 3.1.

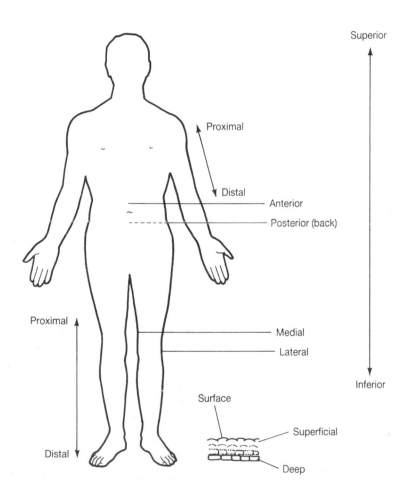

Figure 3.2 *Surfaces of the body*

Table 3.1 *Terminology used to describe the structures of the body*

Description of surface or structure	Position
Anterior or ventral	a surface that faces forwards; a structure that is further forwards than another
Posterior or dorsal	a surface that faces backwards; a structure that is further back than another
Medial	a surface or structure that is nearer to the mid-line than another
Lateral	a surface or structure that is further away from the mid-line than another
Proximal	a structure that is towards the root or origin, i.e. nearer the trunk
Distal	a structure that is further away from the root or origin, i.e. further away from the trunk
Superficial	a structure that is nearer the surface than others
Deep	a structure that lies beneath others, i.e. is further from the surface
Superior	a structure higher than others, i.e. towards the head
Inferior	a structure lower than others

The skeletal system

THE FUNCTIONS OF THE SKELETAL SYSTEM

- Support – the bony framework gives shape to the body, supports the soft tissues and provides attachment for muscles.
- Protection – the bony framework protects delicate internal organs from injury. For example, the brain is protected by the skull, the heart and lungs are protected by the rib cage.
- Movement – is produced by a system of bones, joints and muscles. The bones act as levers and muscles pull on the bones, resulting in movement at the joints.
- Storage of minerals – bones store many minerals, particularly calcium and phosphorus.
- Storage of energy – fats or lipids stored in the yellow bone marrow provide energy when required.
- Storage of tissue that forms blood cells – special connective tissue called red bone marrow produces blood cells. This is found in the spongy bone of the pelvis, vertebrae, ribs, sternum and skull and the ends of the femur and humerus.

THE STRUCTURE OF BONE

Bone is classified as a connective tissue. There are two types of bone tissue, *compact bone* and *cancellous* or *spongy bone*:

- Compact bone is a hard dense tissue which forms the outer layer of bones and gives them strength.
- Cancellous bone forms the inner mass of bones: its spongy structure makes the bones lighter.

Bone is a very hard connective tissue, consisting of cells, collagen fibres and a matrix or ground substance. The matrix is impregnated with mineral salts such as calcium carbonate and calcium phosphate. As these salts are laid down the tissue calcifies and hardens. Bone is a flexible living tissue and has the capacity to repair if damaged.

Various type of bone fracture may occur as a result of injuries sustained in sport, athletics, dance or exercise. Sufficient time must be allowed for calcium salts to be laid down to heal the fracture before pressure is put on the bone.

TYPES OF BONE

There are four different types of bone, named according to their shape:

- Long bones are longer than their width, e.g. femur, tibia, fibula, humerus, radius, ulna, metacarpals, phalanges.
- Short bones of almost equal width and length, e.g. carpal and tarsal bones.
- Flat bones are flat thin bones, found where protection is needed and also where a broad surface is required for the attachment of muscles, e.g. skull bones, scapulae, sternum, ribs.
- Irregular bones are all the bones with complex shapes that do not fit into the above categories, e.g. vertebrae, sacrum, innominate bone, sphenoid, ethmoid.

Other small bones found in the body but not named according to shape are called sesamoid bones: small rounded bones that develop within tendons, such as the patella. They enable the tendon to move smoothly over the underlying bone.

The bones of the skeletal system

It is difficult to study and visualise bones simply by using diagrams. It is easier to learn and much more interesting when a model skeleton and model bones are used. These can be examined and the important features identified and related to one's own body. Only the important and relevant features have been included in the following text. The bones are clearly labelled for easy learning. However, remember to identify the features on model bones and palpate (feel) on your own body where possible.

The human skeleton is made up of 206 bones. These are grouped into two main divisions: the *axial skeleton*, which forms the core or axis of the body, and the *appendicular skeleton*, which forms the girdles and limbs.

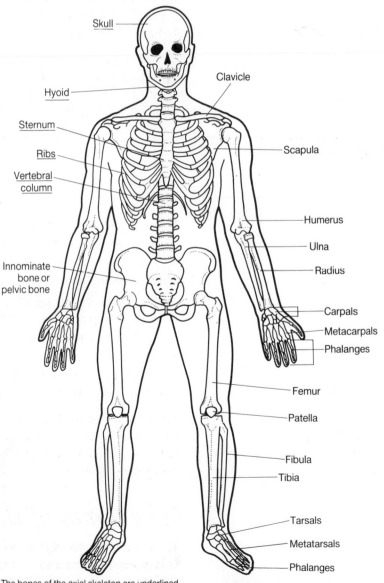

Figure 3.3 *The human skeleton*

The bones of the axial skeleton are underlined

THE AXIAL SKELETON AND THE APPENDICULAR SKELETON

The bones of the axial skeleton are the skull (head), the vertebral column (spine), the sternum (breast bone), the ribs, the hyoid bone (small bone in neck below mandible). The bones of the appendicular skeleton are as shown in Table 3.2.

See figure 3.3

Table 3.2 *The bones of the appendicular skeleton*

Upper limb bones	*Lower limb bones*
Clavicle (collar bone)	Innominate/pelvic bone (hip bone)
Scapula (shoulder bone)	Femur (thigh bone)
Humerus (upper arm bone)	Patella (knee cap)
Radius (forearm – lateral)	Tibia (lower leg – medial)
Ulna (forearm – medial)	Fibula (lower leg – lateral)
Carpals (wrist)	Tarsals (ankle)
Metacarpals (palm)	Metatarsals (foot)
Phalanges (fingers)	Phalanges (toes)

THE BONES OF THE SKULL

These include the cranial and facial bones.

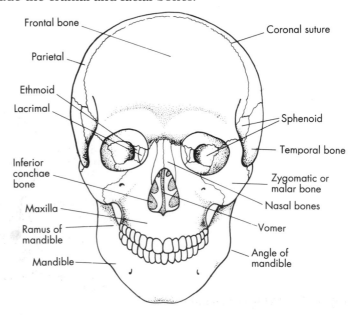

Figure 3.4 *The bones of the skull*

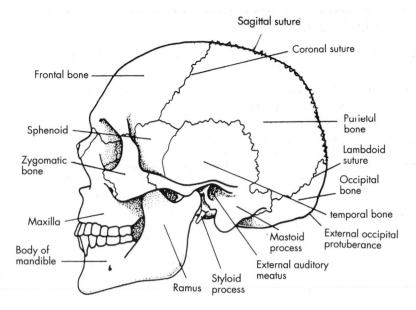

Figure 3.5 *Lateral view of the skull*

There are eight cranial bones: one frontal, two parietal bones, one occipital, two temporal, one sphenoid and one ethmoid.

In addition, there are fourteen facial bones: two lacrimal, two nasal bones, one vomer, two inferior nasal conchae or turbinate bones, two zygomatic bones, two palatine bones, two maxillae and one mandible.

THE SUTURES OF THE SKULL

These are the joints between the bones of the skull. They are immovable fibrous joints. There are four main sutures: coronal, sagittal, lambdoidal and squamous.

THE FEATURES OF THE SKELETAL BONES

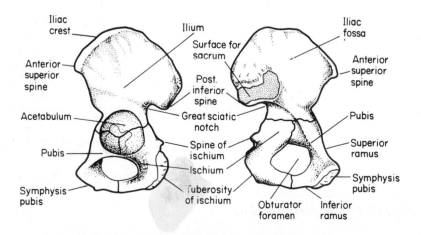

Figure 3.6 *The left innominate bone*

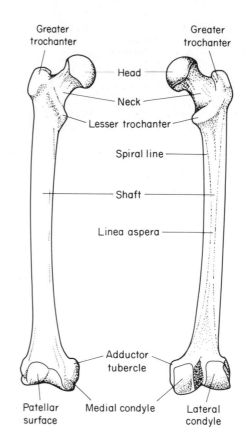

Figure 3.7 *Anterior and posterior views of the right femur*

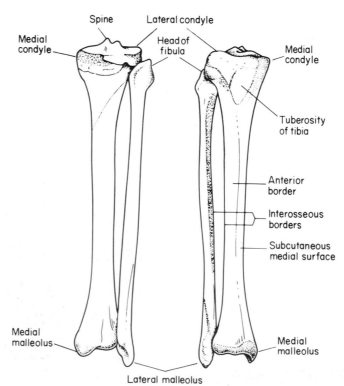

Figure 3.8 *Posterior and anterior views of the tibia and fibula*

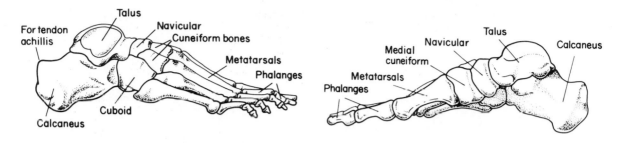

Figure 3.9a, b *The bones of the foot*

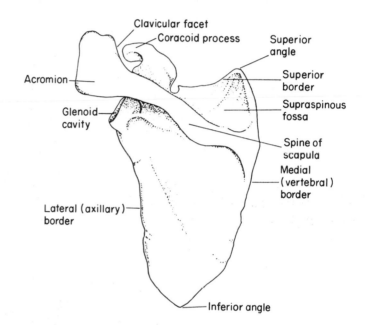

Figure 3.10 *The posterior surface of the scapula*

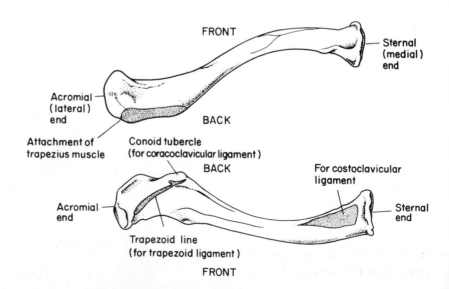

Figure 3.11 *The left clavicle*

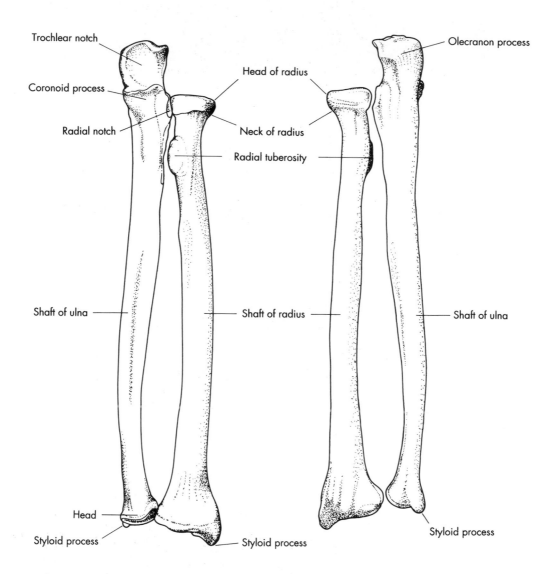

Trochlear notch

Coronoid process

Radial notch

Head of radius

Neck of radius

Radial tuberosity

Olecranon process

Shaft of ulna

Shaft of radius

Shaft of ulna

Head

Styloid process

Styloid process

Styloid process

Figure 3.12 *The left radius and ulna*

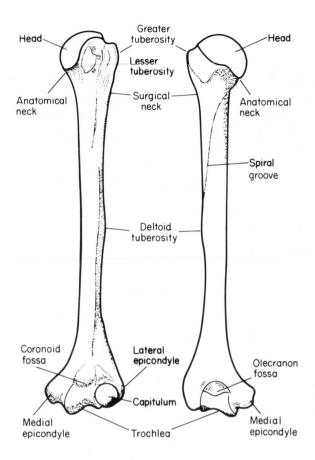

Figure 3.13 *The left humerus*

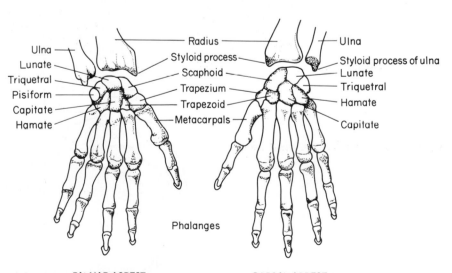

Figure 3.14 *The left hand*   PALMAR ASPECT   DORSAL ASPECT

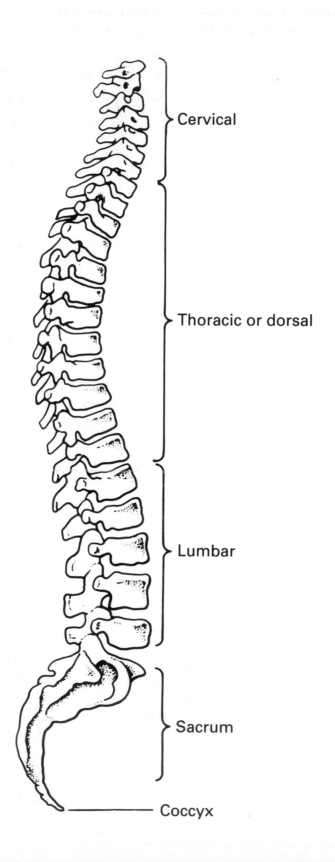

Cervical

Thoracic or dorsal

Lumbar

Sacrum

Coccyx

Figure 3.15 *The vertebral column*

THE VERTEBRAL COLUMN (SPINAL COLUMN)

The vertebral column is composed of 33 vertebrae. Some are fused together, so that in fact there are only 26 bones.

The column is divided into five regions:

- *Cervical* – seven vertebrae (neck)
- *Thoracic* – twelve vertebrae (upper back)
- *Lumbar* – five vertebrae (small of back)
- *Sacral* – five fused vertebrae (sacrum)
- *Coccygeal* – four fused vertebrae (coccyx).

THE FUNCTIONS OF THE VERTEBRAL COLUMN

- It allows movement forward, backward and laterally.
- It protects the spinal cord.
- It supports the head.
- It provides rigidity to maintain the upright posture.
- It provides posterior attachment for the ribs.
- It provides attachment for muscles.
- It acts as a shock absorber.
- The cancellous bone of the vertebrae stores red bone marrow, which forms blood cells.
- It stores minerals.
- It provides the fulcrum for numerous movements.

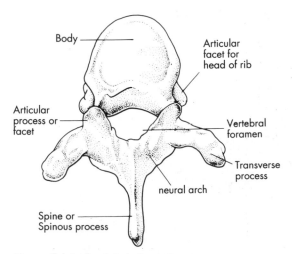

Figure 3.16a, b *(a) A thoracic vertebra*

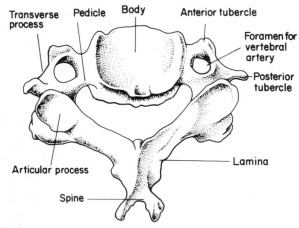

(b) A cervical vertebra

A TYPICAL VERTEBRA

A typical vertebra is composed of several major parts:

- the *body* – a mass of cancellous bone surrounded by a thin layer of compact bone. Body weight is transmitted through these bodies and the inter-vertebral discs that lie between them;

- the *neural or vertebral arch* – a strong arch of bone enclosing the vertebral foramen. It is made up of several fused parts. It protects the spinal cord, which passes down from the brain through the vertebral foramen;

- the *spinous process* – a spikelike backward projection. It provides attachment for many muscles and ligaments;

- the *transverse process* – two projections, one on either side. They also provide attachment for muscles and ligaments;

- four *facets* – surfaces (two above and two below) for articulating with the adjacent vertebrae.

Spaces between the vertebrae known as the *inter-vertebral foramina* allow the passage of nerves entering and leaving the spinal cord along its length.

All vertebrae except the first and second cervical (atlas and axis) have these features in common, but they vary in size, becoming larger lower down for weight bearing. The fused vertebrae of the sacrum and coccyx also differ.

THE INTER-VERTEBRAL DISCS

These lie between the bodies of the vertebrae; they act as shock absorbers and allow for compression and distortion along the column. The core of the disc is the *nucleus pulposus*, which is a jelly-like material consisting of 85 per cent water. Surrounding this is the *annulus fibrosus*, which is composed of many rings of elastic fibres woven at angles to each other. It is thus able to expand and move to absorb compression forces.

As we grow older, the nucleus loses its water-binding capacity, fibro-cartilage replaces the gelatinous substance and the nucleus

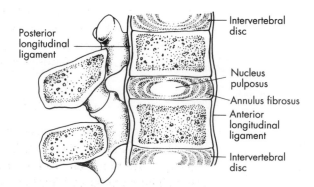

Figure 3.17 *A section through the vertebral column*

gradually hardens. The annulus fibrosus also loses its elasticity. As elasticity and flexibility are lost, the hardened rigid disc becomes more susceptible to injury. If the compression forces are abnormally strong or sudden, the annulus fibrosus may tear or rupture, allowing the nucleus to protrude into the space. This is known as a 'slipped disc' or disc prolapse. If this protrusion presses against a nerve as it passes out of the spinal canal through the inter-vertebral foramen, then neurological symptoms will be felt along the path of the nerve, for example pain, tingling, pins and needles, numbness.

Disc problems can occur at any time, but the likelihood increases as we get older. It is therefore extremely important to consider the age and medical condition of clients when giving any neck and trunk exercises. Failure to do so can result in very serious injury.

MOVEMENT OF THE SPINAL COLUMN

The vertebrae and discs are bound together by strong, powerful ligaments. There is very little movement between adjacent vertebrae, but the total combined movement along the whole length allows considerable movement of the trunk. The movements of the vertebral column are flexion, extension, side flexion and rotation. There is a greater range of movement in the cervical and lumbar regions than in the thoracic. These variations are due to the length and direction of the spinous processes, the ratio between the height of the discs and the height of the vertebral body, and the tension of the supporting ligaments.

Flexion and extension of the neck occur in the cervical region. Flexion and extension of the trunk occur mainly in the lumbar region. Rotation of the trunk occurs mainly in the thoracic region.

DANGEROUS MOVEMENTS

The most hazardous movement is trunk forward flexion, as this movement takes place mainly in the lumbar spine. About 20 per cent of the movement occurs between the fourth and fifth lumbar vertebrae, and 60 to 70 per cent occurs between the fifth lumbar vertebra and the first sacral vertebra. There is therefore a high risk of damage to this vulnerable area of the lower back. See page 163.

THE CURVES OF THE VERTEBRAL COLUMN

The vertebral column shows curves along its length. These are seen in the cervical, thoracic, lumbar and sacral regions. The thoracic and sacral curves are primary curves, being present before birth. The cervical and lumbar curves are secondary curves and develop after birth. The cervical curve develops when the baby lifts its head, the lumbar curve develops as the baby learns to sit and stand. When viewed posteriorly:

- the cervical curve is concave;
- the thoracic curve is convex;
- the lumbar curve is concave;
- the sacral curve is convex.

SPINAL PROBLEMS

Certain spinal problems result in exaggerated or abnormal spinal curves. When the spine is viewed posteriorly the following curves may be seen:

- *Kyphosis* is an exaggerated thoracic curve with increased convexity and forward flexion.
- *Lordosis* is an exaggerated lumbar curve with increased concavity and extension.
- *Kypho-lordosis* is a combination of the above.
- *Scoliosis* is a lateral deviation of the spine. It may deviate to the right or to the left and may show a long C curve or an S curve.

These curves are accompanied by muscle imbalance: some muscles will be too tight and the opposite groups will be over-stretched. Exercises can help to correct these problems.

These problems are fully discussed in chapter 9.

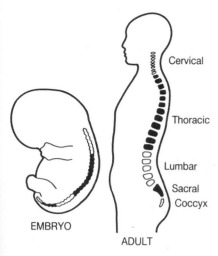

Figure 3.18 *Vertebral curves in the embryo and adult*

T A S K S

Work with a partner.

- Examine your partner's back and identify the five regions of the vertebral column.
- Run your index finger firmly down the spinous processes, leaving a red line. If the line deviates to the right or left it indicates a spinal problem. Name this spinal problem.
- Perform all the movements of the vertebral column.

THE THORAX OR THORACIC CAVITY

This is the bony cage of the chest, composed of the sternum, the 24 ribs and the twelve thoracic vertebrae.

THE STERNUM

The sternum or breast bone is a flat narrow bone made up of three parts:

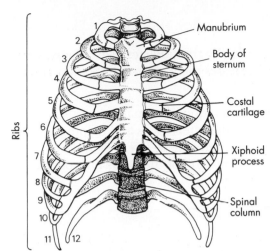

Figure 3.19 *Skeleton of the thorax*

- the *manubrium* – the top part, squarish in shape;
- the *body* – the long middle part;
- the *xiphoid process* – the small pointed lower end.

THE RIBS

The ribs are narrow flat bones articulating with the thoracic vertebrae behind and with the sternum in front. The ribs are arranged in pairs, one on the right and the other on the left:

- Seven pairs are true ribs, which join the sternum.
- Five pairs are false ribs, which join the rib above. Two of these are called floating ribs as they have no attachment in front.

Each rib is joined to the sternum or to the adjacent ribs by a strip of hyaline cartilage. These are called the costal cartilages.

Small muscles known as the 'intercostal muscles' fill the spaces between the ribs. They lie in two layers: eleven internal intercostals and eleven external intercostals on each side of the chest. A large muscle called the diaphragm forms the floor of the thoracic cavity. The lungs lie within and are protected by the thoracic cavity.

THE MECHANISM OF BREATHING

The capacity of the thorax must increase so that air can be taken in and then must decrease so that air can be forced out. During inspiration (breathing in), the intercostal muscles contract and swing the ribs upwards and outwards; the sternum is pushed forwards, and the diaphragm moves downwards. Thus the capacity of the thorax increases sideways, forwards and downwards and the pressure inside the thorax is lowered. When the pressure is reduced below atmospheric pressure (i.e. the pressure of the air outside the body), air rushes in and fills the lungs. Oxygen passes into the bloodstream through the walls of the capillaries surrounding the lungs and carbon dioxide passes the other way. During expiration (breathing out) the intercostal muscles relax, the diaphragm moves upwards, the ribs and sternum collapse back and the lungs recoil. This increases the pressure in the lungs and air is forced out.

During exercise, more oxygen is required to maintain energy for muscle contraction. Therefore the intercostals and diaphragm work harder and as a result they improve in strength and condition. The elasticity and condition of the lungs improves in the same way.

T A S K S

- Place your hands on the sides of the lower ribs. Breathe in deeply and feel the ribs moving outwards and upwards. Breathe out and feel the ribs moving back. Repeat six times.

- Repeat this procedure with the hands over:
  a) the front of the midriff – breathe in and the abdomen moves out; breathe out
  b) the body of the sternum – breathe in and the sternum swings forward; breathe out.

THE GIRDLES

There are two girdles, the pelvic girdle and the shoulder girdle.

THE PELVIC GIRDLE (OR PELVIS)

This is the circle of bone commonly called the hips. It protects various organs, for example the uterus and bladder, and transmits body weight to the legs. It is shaped rather like a basin and has an inner and outer surface.

The pelvic girdle is made up of three bones – two innominate bones and the sacrum (part of the vertebral column).

The two large innominate or pelvic bones articulate in front at a cartilaginous joint called the 'pubic symphysis'. At the back they articulate on each side of the sacrum at gliding synovial joints called the 'sacro-iliac joints'. There is hardly any movement at these joints as they fit tightly together and are held in place by very strong ligaments. The pelvis is supported on the femoral heads and may tilt forward, backward or sideways. Pelvic tilt accompanies movements of the trunk and hip joints, as is shown in chapter 4.

THE SHOULDER GIRDLE (THE PECTORAL GIRDLE)

The shoulder girdle is composed of two clavicles in front and two scapulae at the back. Anteriorly, each clavicle articulates with the

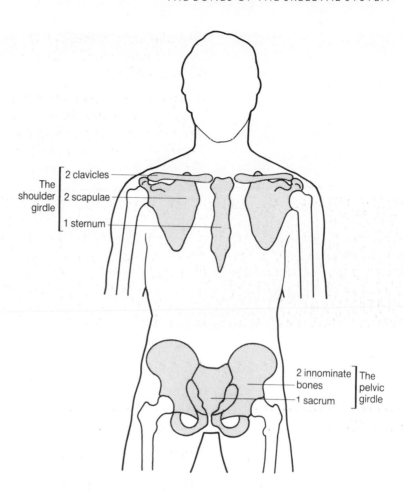

Figure 3.20 *Shoulder and pelvic girdles*

sternum at the sterno-clavicular joint. Laterally, the clavicles articulate with the acromion process of the scapula at the acromio-clavicular joint.

The shoulder girdle forms an incomplete ring of bone around the upper thorax, joining the upper limbs to the axial skeleton.

Movement of the shoulder girdle accompanies movements of the shoulder joint. These movements of the girdle allow a far greater range of arm movements.

QUESTIONS

1 Compare the two main divisions of the human skeleton.
2 List the bones in each division.
3 Explain the functions of the skeletal system.
4 Explain why cancellous bone is sometimes known as spongy bone.
5 List the four main types of bones and give one example of each.
6 Describe the anatomical position.
7 Define the following terms:
   a   anterior surface
   b   proximal end
   c   medial
   d   superior structure
   e   deep muscle
8 List the bones of the skull.
9 Name the regions of the vertebral column and give the number of vertebrae in each.
10 Give two functions of the inter-vertebral discs.
11 Compare the following spinal problems: kyphosis, lordosis, scoliosis.
12 List the bones that form the thoracic cavity or thorax.
13 Where is the xiphoid process located?
14 Explain the terms true and false ribs.
15 Label the diagram below:

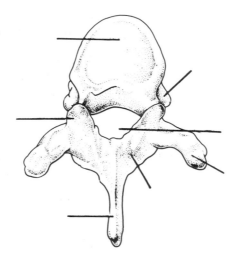

Figure 3.21. *A typical vertebra*

CHAPTER 4

The joints of the skeletal system

Joints

When two or more bones meet they form a joint, sometimes called an articulation. All body movement occurs at joints, from the small movements of the fingers to the large movements of the shoulder. The bones are held together by connective tissue and are moved by the contraction of skeletal muscle.

The shape of the articulating bones and the flexibility and tensile strength of the surrounding connective tissue determines the strength, stability and movement of joints.

Bones with curved surfaces that fit into each other and are close together form strong stable joints with less movement. Bones with little curvature that fit together loosely form joints that are less stable but allow greater movement.

The terminology of joint movement

The following terms are used to describe the direction of joint movement:

- *flexion* – the bringing together of two surfaces (a bending movement), (e.g. bending the elbow or knee);
- *extension* – movement in the opposite direction to flexion (a straightening movement), (e.g. straightening the elbow or knee);
- *abduction* – movement away from the mid-line (e.g. taking the arm away from the body);
- *adduction* – movement towards the mid-line (e.g. taking the arm back to the body);
- *rotation* – movement around a long axis, which may be medial rotation (e.g. turning the arm in) or lateral rotation (e.g. turning the arm out);

- *circumduction* – a movement where the limb describes a cone whose apex lies in the joint: a combination of flexion, abduction, extension and adduction (e.g. circling the shoulder joint or hip joint round and round).

Movements that occur between the radius and ulna:

- *supination* turns the hand forwards or upwards;
- *pronation* turns the hand backwards or downwards.

Movements of the ankle joint:

- *dorsi-flexion* – pulling the foot upwards;
- *plantar flexion* – pointing the foot downwards.

Movements of the foot (occurring between the tarsal joints):

- *inversion* – turning the sole of the foot inwards;
- *eversion* – turning the sole of the foot outwards.

Movements of the shoulder girdle (and jaw):

- *elevation* – lifting the shoulder (jaw) upwards;
- *depression* – dropping the shoulders (jaw);
- *protraction* – drawing the shoulders (jaw) forward;
- *retraction* – drawing the shoulders (jaw) backwards.

Movements of the head and trunk:

- *forward flexion* – bending the head or trunk forward;
- *side flexion* – bending the head or trunk to the side. It may be right side flexion or left side flexion;
- *extension* – moving the head or trunk backwards;
- *rotation* – turning the head or trunk to the right or to the left, a twisting movement;
- *circumduction* – moving the head or trunk in a circular motion.

The terminology used to describe joint movement must be understood. Learning these thoroughly now makes muscle work much easier later on.

Some joints only move in two directions, for example the elbow and knee, whilst others will move in six directions, for example the shoulder and hip joints. As has previously been mentioned, muscles pull on the bones to produce these movements. Therefore some muscles will be *flexors*, producing flexion at the joint, whilst other muscles will be *extensors*, producing extension at the joint, and so on. When one group of muscles contracts to produce movement (the agonists) the opposite groups must relax to allow the movement to take place (the antagonists). See page 83.

The classification of joints

There are three main groups:

- *Fibrous* joints are immovable. The bones fit tightly together and are held firmly by fibrous tissue. There is no joint cavity. Examples are the sutures of the skull.

- *Cartilaginous* joints are slightly movable. The bones are connected by a disc of fibro-cartilage. There is no joint cavity. Examples are the symphysis pubis (between the pubic bones) and the inter-vertebral joints (between the vertebral bodies).

- *Synovial* joints are freely movable. These are the most numerous in the body. There are six different types of synovial joints. They are classified according to their planes of movement, which depend on the shape of the articulating bones. All the freely movable joints of the body are synovial joints and although their shape and movements vary, they all have certain characteristics in common.

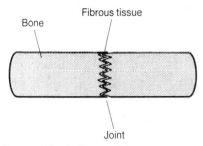

Figure 4.1 *A fibrous joint*

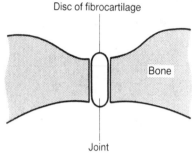

Figure 4.2 *A cartilaginous joint*

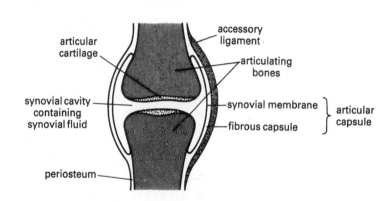

Figure 4.3 *A synovial joint*

FEATURES OF A TYPICAL SYNOVIAL JOINT

- A joint cavity (space within the joint)

- Hyaline cartilage, which covers the surfaces of the articulating bones. Sometimes called articular cartilage, it reduces friction and allows smooth movement. As previously mentioned, with age, injury or disease there may be erosion or damage of this cartilage. Friction will increase as bone moves over bone, the joint will be stiff and movements painful. Regular exercise will delay the onset of these problems, but if there is joint damage exercises must only be performed under medical supervision

- The capsule or articulating capsule, which surrounds the joint like a sleeve. It holds the bones together and encloses the cavity. The capsule is strengthened on the outside by ligaments, which help to stabilise and strengthen the joints. Ligaments may also be found inside a joint, holding the bones together in order to increase stability. The movement at any joint will be limited by the tightness or rigidity of the capsule and ligaments. Flexibility exercises and full-range mobility exercises will maintain and increase the extensibility of these structures and maintain full-range joint movement

- The synovial membrane lining the capsule, which produces synovial fluid
- Synovial fluid or synovium, a viscous fluid which lubricates and nourishes the joint. Regular exercise stimulates an increase in the production of synovial fluid, so that lubrication and nourishment of the cartilage is increased

DISCS (MENISCI)

Some joints, such as the knee, have pads of fibro-cartilage called discs. They are attached to the bones and give the joint a better 'fit'. They also cushion movement. These structures are prone to damage and tearing, usually as a result of excessive stress and rotational forces.

BURSAE

Any movement produces friction between the moving parts. In order to reduce friction, sac-like structures containing synovial fluid are found between tissues. These are called *bursae* and are usually found between tendons and bone. They may become inflamed following injury or repetitive stress. This results in swelling, stiffness and pain of the joint.

CLASSIFICATION OF THE SIX SYNOVIAL JOINTS

Table 4.1   *The synovial joints*

Type of joint	*Examples*	*Movements*
Gliding joints	intercarpal and intertarsal joints	multiaxial; movements limited to gliding or shifting
Hinge joints	elbow, knee, ankle, interphalangeal joints (joints of fingers and toes)	uniaxial and one plane only (sagittal plane, frontal axis); movements – flexion and extension
Pivot joints	superior radio-ulnar joint and atlas on axis (moves the head left and right)	uniaxial and one plane only (horizontal plane, vertical axis); movement – rotation
Ellipsoid (condyloid) joints	wrist (radio-carpal), knuckle (metacarpo-phalangeal joint)	biaxial and in two planes (frontal and sagittal axes, sagittal and frontal planes); movements – flexion, extension, adduction, abduction, circumduction

Saddle joints	carpo-metacarpal joint of thumb (base of thumb)	multiaxial – sagittal, frontal and vertical axes with corresponding planes; movements – flexion, extension, adduction, abduction, rotation (limited), circumduction
Ball and socket joints	hip and shoulder joints	multiaxial – sagittal, frontal and vertical axes with corresponding planes; movements – flexion, extension, adduction, abduction, rotation (medial and lateral), circumduction

The range of movement at joints

The range and degree of movement at joints will vary from individual to individual and will depend on many factors. An understanding of these factors will enable the therapist to plan realistic objectives and avoid being over-ambitious.

- *The shape and contour of the articulating surfaces.* The range of movement will be limited when the bones fit tightly into each other. Examine the hip and shoulder joints: both are synovial ball and socket joints capable of the same number of movements, but the shoulder joint allows a far greater range than the hip joint. This is because the shoulder has a shallow socket (the glenoid cavity) for articulating with the large ball (the head of the humerus), so the movement is not restricted by the depth of the socket. The hip, on the other hand, has a deep socket (acetabulum) into which the head of the femur fits tightly and securely.

- *The tension of the connective tissue components* – the capsule and the ligaments supporting the joint. Ligaments are made of tough, non-elastic, white fibrous tissue. They are found strengthening the capsule around the outside of joints and sometimes inside the joints. They hold the bones together to stabilise and support the joint. They are particularly important for loosely-fitting joints such as the shoulder and weight-bearing joints such as the knee. These ligaments prevent abnormal movements, but if a joint is pushed beyond its range with great enough force these ligaments may tear. Ligaments may be partially torn, as in sprains, or they may rupture completely and the joint may dislocate.

- *The tension of muscles and tendons around the joint.* Tight muscles will limit the movement in underlying joints. Cold muscles are not as extensible as warm muscles and their tension may prevent full joint movement. Forcing a joint when the muscles around it are cold may result in tears or strains of the muscle fibres. It is therefore important to perform warm-up routines before exercising joints through their full range. Some muscles, such as the hamstrings, pass over two joints and the position of one joint limits movement in the other. Note the difference in the range of movement when flexing the hip with the knee straight and flexing the hip with the knee bent. The range of movement is far greater in the latter.

- *The approximation of soft tissue near the joint.* Joint movement is limited when surfaces come into contact with each other, preventing further movement, for example, flexion of the elbow joint is limited when the muscles of the forearm touch the biceps.

- *Ageing* will affect joint range. Children are more supple than young adults, and the young adults more supple than the elderly, because tissues and ligaments tighten with age. Good regular exercise routines will help to maintain range. So called double-jointed people have a greater range of joint movement because they are born with lax ligaments.

Because of the importance of joint movements in exercises, the basic structure and movements of each joint must be clearly understood. This knowledge enables the therapist to select appropriate exercises to maintain range and mobility and, most importantly, to give advice on the prevention of injury, i.e. strains, sprains, dislocation and fractures.

The four ranges of movement are fully discussed in chapter 7.

The major features of skeletal joints

TASKS

- Examine diagrams 4.4–4.9 and learn the major features.
- Examine models of joints and identify the major features.
- Relate each joint to your own body and perform the possible movement.
- Working in pairs, ask your partner to perform named movements, such as flexion of the hip joint or extension of the knee joint.

THE HIP JOINT

Type: Synovial – ball and socket
Bones: The head of the femur articulates with the
              acetabulum of the innominate bone

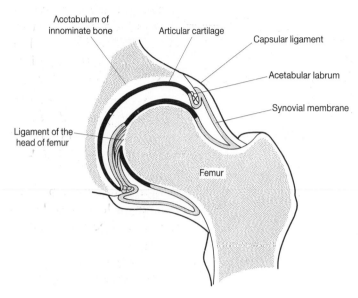

Acetabulum of
innominate bone   Articular cartilage
                                            Capsular ligament

                                            Acetabular labrum

                                            Synovial membrane

Ligament of the
head of femur

                                    Femur

Figure 4.4 *The hip joint*

Movements: Flexion, extension (sagittal plane)
              Abduction, adduction (frontal plane)
              Rotation (medial and lateral) (horizontal plane)
              Circumduction (a combination of flexion
              abduction, extension and adduction).

True flexion and extension of the hip joint are limited to 90°
flexion and only 10° extension, but these movements are greatly
increased by tilting and rotation of the pelvis forwards and
backwards and by associated movements of the vertebral column.

THE KNEE JOINT

Type: Synovial – hinge
Bones: The condyles of the femur articulate with the
              condyles of the tibia. (The posterior aspect of the
              patella also articulates)
Movements: Flexion and extension (sagittal plane). In flexion
              there is slight rotation

The knee joint is susceptible to many injuries as its stability
depends on its powerful ligaments and muscles. Severe stresses can

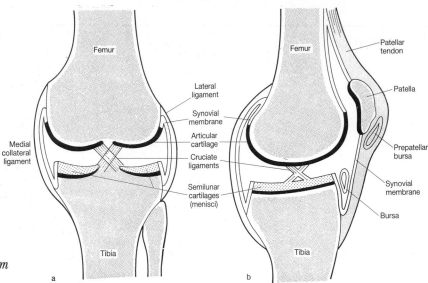

Figure 4.5a, b *The knee joint (a) viewed from the front (b) viewed from the side*

cause sprains, tears or ruptures of any of the ligaments, i.e. the medial and lateral collateral ligaments or the cruciate ligaments. The menisci or cartilages may also be damaged and may require surgical removal.

THE ANKLE JOINT

Type:	Synovial – hinge
Bones:	The malleoli of the tibia and fibula articulate with the talus
Movements:	Plantar flexion – pointing toe down (flexion)
	Dorsi-flexion – pulling foot up (extension)

THE SUBTALAR AND TALO-CALCANEO NAVICULAR JOINTS

Type:	Synovial – gliding
Bones:	Tarsal bones
Movements:	Inversion – turning sole inwards
	Eversion – turning sole outwards

The ligaments around the ankle joint are susceptible to injury, a condition commonly called sprained ankle. The lateral ligament is the most vulnerable as there is a greater range of inversion if the

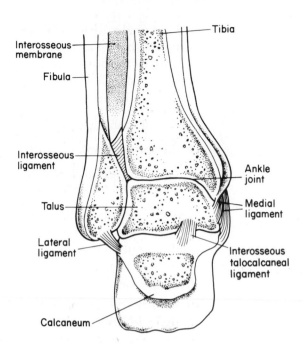

Interosseous membrane

Fibula

Interosseous ligament

Talus

Lateral ligament

Calcaneum

Tibia

Ankle joint

Medial ligament

Interosseous talocalcaneal ligament

Figure 4.6 *The ankle joint*

ankle is forced inward. However, tears of the medial ligament occur in forced eversion injuries. Forced plantar flexion will tear the capsular ligament anteriorly.

THE JOINTS OF THE FOOT

The 26 bones of the foot articulate with each other, forming a variety of joints. The bones of the foot form three arches, which help to absorb shock and prevent jarring during walking, running, etc.

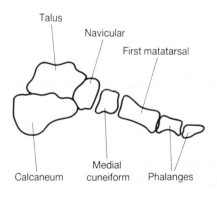

Talus

Navicular

First matatarsal

Calcaneum

Medial cuneiform

Phalanges

Figure 4.7 *The medial arch of the (left) foot*

- The *medial arch* runs along the inside of the foot from the heel (calcaneus) to the three medial toes. This arch is supported by the tendons of the tibialis anterior and tibialis posterior muscles, which act as slings lifting the arch. Normally this arch is not in contact with the ground during weight-bearing. If the muscles and ligaments are weak, the arch drops to create the condition known as flat feet. If the muscles and ligaments are tight the arch is held high, and this is known as high instep.

- The *lateral arch* runs along the outside of the foot from the heel to the two lateral toes. This arch is supported by the tendons of the peroneus longus and peroneus brevis muscles. This is low to the ground and transmits body weight from the heel along the outer border of the foot to the toes during weight-bearing.

- The *anterior transverse arch* lies under the ball of the foot along the metatarsal heads. It is supported by ligaments and the

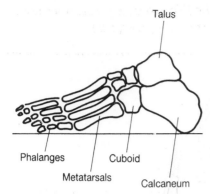

Figure 4.8 *The lateral arch of the (left) foot*

lumbrical muscles. Collapse of this arch can lead to severe pain under the metatarsal heads. Numerous ligaments and small muscles support these bones in the sole of the foot. They are arranged in four layers, and are protected and separated from the skin by the plantar fascia.

Two important ligaments are:

- the spring ligament, which passes from calcaneus to navicular;
- the long plantar ligament, which passes from calcaneus to cuboid and the middle three metatarsals.

The movements of the foot during walking and running are very complex and good foot function is essential to prevent stresses in higher joints. The walking action should begin by striking with the heel, then transfer the weight to the outer border and push off from the toes. The skin over the sole, meanwhile, relays important sensory stimuli to the brain. Impaired foot function can give rise to many problems, such as poor co-ordination, strains on ligaments, stresses at joints and impairment of the function of muscles, with accompanying pain and stiffness. Care of the feet is a priority for everyone partaking in sport and exercise, and choice of footwear is exceedingly important.

THE SHOULDER

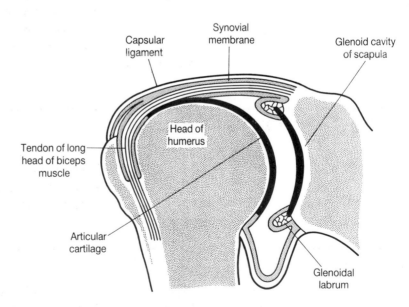

Figure 4.9 *The shoulder joint*

Type: Synovial – ball and socket
Bones: The head of the humerus articulates with the glenoid cavity of the scapula
Movement: Flexion and extension, abduction and adduction, rotation (medial and lateral), circumduction

The range of movement at the shoulder joint is greatly increased by accompanying movements of the shoulder girdle.

The elbow joint

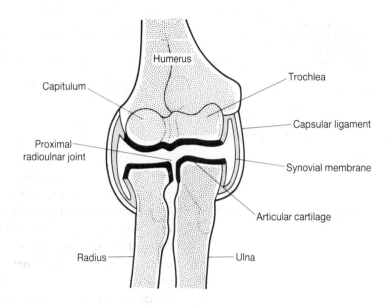

Figure 4.10 *The elbow joint*

Type:	Synovial – hinge joint
Bones:	The trochlea of the humerus articulates with the trochlear notch of the ulna and the head of the radius with the capitulum of the humerus
Movements:	Flexion and extension

The superior radio-ulnar joint

Type:	Synovial – pivot
Bones:	The head of the radius articulates with the radial notch of the ulna
Movements:	Pronation and supination

The wrist joint

Type:	Synovial – ellipsoid (condyloid)
Bones:	The lower end of the radius and disc of the ulna articulate with the scaphoid, lunate and triquetral
Movements:	Flexion and extension, abduction and adduction, circumduction

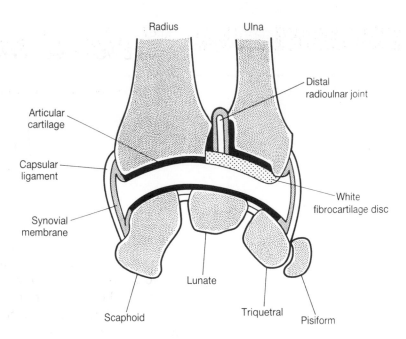

Figure 4.11 *The wrist joint*

QUESTIONS

1 Define the term *articulation*.

2 List the three main groups of joints and give an example from each group.

3 Give the functions of the following parts of a synovial joint:
  a   the synovial membrane
  b   the synovial fluid
  c   the hyaline cartilage.

4 Name one joint where discs or menisci are to be found.

5 List the six types of synovial joint.

6 Briefly explain any four factors that limit the range of movement at joints.

7 List and define the movements of the hip joint.

8 Give two reasons why there is a greater range of movement in the shoulder joint compared with the hip joint, although both are ball and socket.

9 Give the movements of the ankle joint (remember that this is a hinge joint).

10 Name and describe the arches of the foot.

11 Describe the action of walking.

12 Name and describe the movements that occur between the radius and ulna.

CHAPTER 5

Skeletal muscle

Muscles form the body flesh. Their functions are to produce movement, to maintain posture and to produce body heat. Muscle tissue is totally under the control of the nervous system: impulses transmitted from the brain via motor nerves initiate contraction of the muscle fibres. This contraction pulls on the bones and movement occurs at the joints.

The structure of skeletal muscle

Skeletal muscle is composed of muscle fibres arranged in bundles called fasciculi; many bundles of fibres make up the complete muscle. The fibres, bundles and muscles are surrounded and protected by connective tissue sheaths:

- The connective tissue around each fibre is called the *endomysium.*
- The connective tissue around each bundle is called the *perimysium.*
- The connective tissue around the muscle is called the *epimysium.*

MUSCLE FIBRES

Muscle fibres are long, thin multi-nucleate cells. The fibres vary from ten to 100 microns in diameter and from a few millimetres to many centimetres in length. The long fibres extend the full length of the muscle, while the short fibres end in connective tissue intersections within the muscle.

Each muscle fibre is bound by a cell membrane known as the *sarcolemma,* just beneath which lie the nuclei. The cytoplasm of the muscle cell is known as the *sarcoplasm.* It contains large numbers of mitochondria and other organelles. Muscle fibres are made up of smaller protein threads called *myofibrils.* These run the whole length of the fibre and are the elements which contract and relax. Myofibrils are made up of even smaller threads called *myofilaments.*

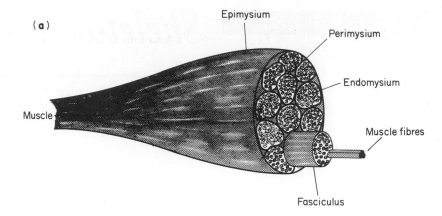

Figure 5.1a *(a) The structure of skeletal muscle*

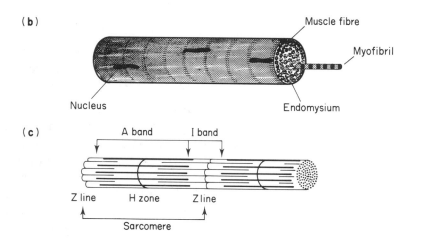

Figure 5.1b, c *(b) Single muscle fibre, showing characteristic striations (c) Myofibril, illustrating a sarcomere*

Under an electron microscope, myofibrils are seen to have alternate light and dark bands called I and A bands. In the middle of the dark A band is a lighter zone, the H zone. In the middle of the light I band is a dark line, the Z line.

The segment between two Z lines is known as the *sarcomere.* These sarcomeres are repeated along the whole length of the myofibril. Each sarcomere contains overlapping thick and thin myofilaments. The thin myofilaments are made of the protein *actin.* They begin at the Z line and extend into the A band, where they overlap with the thick myofilaments, which are made of the protein *myosin.* These thick bands have small cross-bridges projecting sideways towards active sites on the thin bands. These are very important: when a stimulus from the nervous system is received by the muscle fibre, a series of chemical reactions takes place which results in the cross-bridges linking and pulling the thin bands towards the thick bands. The sliding thin bands pull on the Z lines and each sarcomere shortens. Consequently, the myofibrils and fibres shorten and the whole muscle contracts. The energy for this contraction is obtained from the breakdown of ATP (adenosine triphosphate) stored in the myosine cross-bridges.

Figure 5.2a, b *The sarcomere (a) during relaxation (b) during contraction*

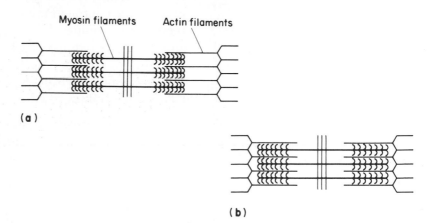

Muscle relaxation occurs when no stimulus is received from the nervous system. The thin bands slide back to their precontracted state and the muscle relaxes.

Muscle elongation only occurs as a result of some pulling force on the muscle. This force may be the pull of antagonistic muscles (i.e. on the opposite side of the joint), the pull of gravity, the pull of weights, springs, etc., or manual pulling by oneself or another person. The fibres elongate because the thin filaments move away from the thick filaments and each sarcomere gets longer. The pull must allow at least one cross-bridge to remain intact; otherwise, the sarcomere will rupture. Strong forces can cause small tears within a muscle because the cross-bridges are no longer intact. During exercise and sports, excessive stress may result in muscle tears.

MUSCLE FIBRE TYPES

A muscle is composed of different types of muscle fibres. Some fibres rely on aerobic energy systems, while others rely on anaerobic energy systems, as we shall see later. The proportion of each type of fibre within the muscle will vary depending on the function of the muscle.

● Slow twitch fibres or slow oxidative fibres (red fibres) are capable of sustaining tension for long periods of time. They contract slowly but can contract repeatedly over long periods. They are recruited for endurance activities such as marathon running, jogging, swimming, the maintenance of posture and aerobic exercise. They have high-density capillary networks and are well supplied with blood. They have high levels of oxidative enzymes and myoglobin, which stores oxygen until it is needed by the mitochondria for generating ATP. Contraction utilises aerobic metabolism.

- Fast twitch fibres or fast glycolytic fibres (white fibres), on the other hand, contract rapidly but fatigue easily. They are recruited intermittently for short periods when bursts of speed and power are required, such as 100 and 200 metre sprints, the push-off from starting blocks, squash and all fast movements. They have high levels of glycogen and glycolytic enzymes. Contraction utilises anaerobic metabolism.

Human muscle contains both types of fibres in varying proportions and they are recruited for different activities.

In some animals these fibres are clearly defined, for example in chickens, where the red fibres are found in the postural muscles of the legs and the white fibres in the breasts and wings, where more rapid action is required for flying.

MUSCLE SHAPE

Muscle shape varies depending on the function of the muscle. The fleshy bulk of the muscle is known as the belly. The bundles of muscle fibres lie either parallel or obliquely to the line of pull of the muscle. Parallel fibres are found in strap-like and fusiform muscles. These long fibres allow for a wide range of movement. The shorter oblique fibres are found in triangular and pennate muscles, where muscle strength is required.

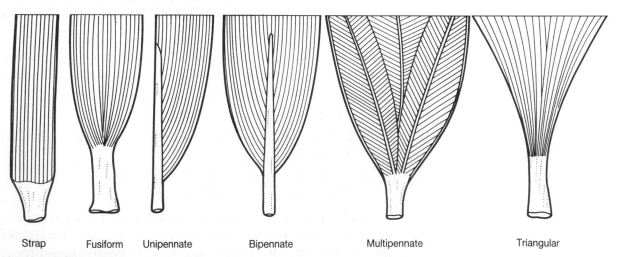

Strap   Fusiform   Unipennate   Bipennate   Multipennate   Triangular

Figure 5.3 *Muscle shape*

The contraction of skeletal muscle

THE 'ALL OR NONE' LAW

Stimuli from the brain and spinal cord are transmitted to a muscle fibre via its motor unit. The motor unit is composed of an anterior horn cell in the spinal cord, its axon, axon branches and the muscle fibres they supply. When skeletal muscle fibres respond to nervous stimuli, the weakest stimulus that produces a contraction is known as the threshold stimulus. The threshold stimulus will produce a contraction of maximum force in the fibres supplied by that motor unit. Fibres do not respond with the partial contraction, they contract with maximum force or not at all. This is known as the 'all or none' law. However, this is not true of the muscle as a whole. Muscle contraction may be weak or strong depending on the number of motor units stimulated. Different types of fibres within a muscle respond to stimuli of different frequencies, so that some will contract while others will not. The strength of muscle contraction will also be affected by lack of nutrients, lack of oxygen or the presence of lactic acid.

MUSCLE ATTACHMENTS

As previously explained, a muscle is composed of muscle fibres and connective tissue components, namely the endomysium, perimysium and epimysium. Certain muscles have connective tissue intersections, dividing the muscle into several bellies, as seen in the rectus abdominus.

Sheets of connective tissue blend at either end of the muscle and attach the muscle to the underlying bones. Muscles are attached by either tendons or aponeuroses to the periosteum, the connective tissue covering the bone.

- *Tendons* are tough cord-like structures of connective tissue which attach muscles to bones.
- *Aponeuroses* are flat sheets of connective tissue which attach muscles along the length of the bone.

A muscle has at least two points of attachment, known as the origin and insertion of the muscle. These are attached on either side of the joint. The origin is usually proximal and stationary or immovable. The insertion is usually distal and movable.

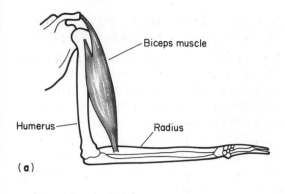

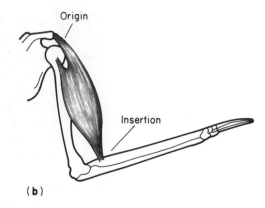

Figure 5.4 *The origin and insertion of a muscle*

When muscles contract, it is usual for the insertion to move towards the origin, which remains stationary; however, certain muscles can also work in reverse, the origin moving towards the insertion. This is known as 'the reverse action of muscles' or 'origin–insertion reversed'. For example, the gluteus maximus extends the hip joint. When it pulls the leg backwards, the insertion on the femur moves towards the origin on the pelvis, which remains stationary. However, if the trunk is in forward flexion, the gluteus maximus can pull the trunk upright: when its origin on the pelvis moves towards the insertion on the femur, which remains stationary (see Figure 5.5).

MUSCLE TONE

Muscle tone is the state of partial contraction or tension found in muscles even when at rest. A small number of muscle fibres will

Figure 5.5 *Actions of the gluteus maximus*
(a) Extension of the hip joint, the insertion moves towards the origin
(b) Raising the trunk, the origin moves towards the insertion

always be in a state of contraction. This is sufficient to produce tautness in the muscle, but not to result in full contraction and movement. Different groups of fibres contract alternately, working a 'shift' system to prevent fatigue of the few. Changes in muscle tone are adjusted according to the information received from sensory receptors within the muscles and their tendons. *Muscle spindles* transmit information on the degree of stretch within the muscle. *Tendon receptors* called Golgi organs transmit information on the amount of tension applied to the tendon by muscle contraction. Too much stretch and tension will be counteracted by a reduction in muscle tone. Too little will be counteracted by an increase in muscle tone. Muscle tone is essential for maintaining upright posture.

- Hypotonic muscles, i.e. those with less than the normal degree of tone, are said to be flaccid.

- Hypertonic muscles, i.e. those with a greater degree of muscle tone and where fibres are over-contracted and rigid, are said to be spastic.

- A contraction that increases muscle tone but does not change the length of the muscle is called isometric contraction (equal length).

- A contraction where muscle tone remains the same but the muscle changes in length is called isotonic contraction (equal tone).

(In practice tone does change through the range, depending on the angle of muscle pull: see chapter 8).

BLOOD SUPPLY TO SKELETAL MUSCLE

A plentiful supply of oxygen and nutrients to produce energy are required by contracting muscles and the waste products of these energy-producing reactions must be removed. The supplies of oxygen and nutrients required by a muscle are brought by the blood via the arteries, and the waste products are removed via the veins. The arteries branch to form smaller arteries and arterioles within the perimysium. They then divide further to form capillary networks within the endomysium, where they join venules, which lead to veins. When muscles are relaxed, the capillary network delivers blood to the muscle fibres. When muscles contract, the pressure impedes the flow of blood through the capillary beds. This reduces the supply of oxygen and nutrients and limits the removal of waste. During exercise, muscle fibres alternately contract and relax and the capillaries deliver blood during the relaxation phase. However, repeated or sustained contraction, such as isometric work or exercising without sufficient rest periods, prevents the flow of blood to the muscle fibres, due to compression on the blood vessels and the capillaries. This results in muscle fatigue due to lack of oxygen and nutrients and the accumulation of waste products such as lactic acid. The strength and speed of contraction become progressively weaker, and as fatigue continues the muscle fails to relax completely, resulting in muscle spasm and pain.

Regardless of the activity, muscles must be given sufficient time to relax completely. This will ensure an adequate blood supply and prevent fatigue. Regular endurance aerobic exercise results in an increase in blood vessels and capillary networks to the muscles. This will improve the blood supply, increase levels of oxygen and nutrients and reduce levels of lactic acid. Thus the capacity to exercise without fatigue will improve.

Energy for muscle contraction

All cells require energy for cellular activity. Muscle cells expend far more energy than other cells: they convert chemical energy into mechanical energy. Energy for muscle contraction is supplied by the chemical compound *adenosine triphosphate* (ATP). The breakdown of ATP releases energy, which triggers the rowing action of the myosine cross-bridges and hence the sliding action of muscle contraction.

A small quantity of ATP is stored within the muscle. When this is used up it must be replenished by the breakdown of stored phosphocreatine (PC) and then by the breakdown of carbohydrates and fats. Carbohydrates are broken down into glucose and then glycogen, which is stored in muscles and in the liver. Excess carbohydrate is converted to fat and stored in adipose tissue. Fats are broken down into fatty acids, stored in adipose tissue and in the blood, and triglycerides, stored in muscle. These are used to produce ATP by chemical reactions in the mitochondria. (Protein is only used for ATP under extreme conditions of starvation or ultra-marathon running.)

Some of these chemical reactions utilise oxygen and are termed aerobic energy systems. Other reactions do not utilise oxygen and are termed anaerobic energy systems.

When muscles are at rest ATP, phosphocreatine, glycogen and triglycerides are stored within the muscle, together with certain enzymes which act as catalysts (a catalyst is a chemical which changes the rate of a reaction but remains unchanged itself).

When a muscle is stimulated to contract, immediate energy is obtained from stored ATP (anaerobic). After five to six seconds of activity the ATP is used up and must be replenished by the breakdown of phosphocreatine. This supplies energy for ten to fifteen seconds, until the supply of phosphocreatine is depleted. This process also takes place without oxygen and is anaerobic.

Further energy is obtained by the breakdown of foodstuffs. The first source of energy is stored glucose (glycogen) and the second source is fatty acids and triglycerides. Glycogen is broken down to a substance called pyruvic acid by a process known as *glycolysis*. The next stage depends on whether there is sufficient oxygen available or not, as described below.

THE ANAEROBIC OR LACTIC ACID SYSTEM

During vigorous exercise, if the cardio-respiratory system is unable to supply oxygen quickly enough to meet the demand of the contracting muscles, pyruvic acid is broken down into lactic acid. This waste product builds up in the muscles and in the blood. The build-up of lactic acid produces fatigue and eventually pain and stiffness. Because there is a shortage of oxygen, an oxygen debt is created which must be repaid at the end of vigorous activity by deep breathing. This system provides energy for short, sharp bursts of activity lasting up to two minutes, such as a quick dash, sprinting or throwing. Eventually, as the oxygen debt is repaid, the lactic acid is converted back to pyruvic acid and broken down into carbon dioxide and water.

THE AEROBIC SYSTEM

During steady-state exercise, sufficient oxygen can be breathed in and delivered to the muscles via the circulation. The pyruvic acid produced by the breakdown of glycogen is oxidised to carbon dioxide and water by a complex series of chemical reactions (known as the Krebs cycle). This system produces far more ATP than the lactic acid system and activity can continue indefinitely, providing there is sufficient oxygen available, as no toxic waste builds up in the muscle.

The aerobic system is used in jogging, swimming, running, cross-country skiing, cycling, aerobic dance and other aerobic exercises. The activity must be steady-state and below maximal effort to allow the systems to deliver and utilise oxygen. This system goes on to use fatty acids and triglycerol for energy once glycogen is depleted. Acute feelings of exhaustion are experienced as glycogen is depleted, as in 'hitting the wall' in marathon running.

All activities begin with the anaerobic ATP–PC phase, and will then move into either the aerobic or the anaerobic system, but the majority of sports will require use of both systems at various points.

Table 5.1 *The three metabolic systems*

Anaerobic (alactic): ATP–PC system	Anaerobic: lactic acid system	Aerobic: oxygen system
Uses stored ATP and PC	Uses glycogen	Uses glycogen, fatty acids, triglycerol
Beginning of all activities and very fast short bursts up to fifteen seconds	Fast activity up to two minutes	Slow steady activity indefinitely
Example: quick dash	Example: 400 metre run	Example: jogging
Contraction stops when ATP and PC are used up	Contraction stops due to lactic acid build-up and creation of oxygen debt	Contraction maintained indefinitely until exhaustion is reached

AEROBIC AND ANAEROBIC EXERCISES

These names are derived from the energy systems used. Most activities involve both aerobic and anaerobic metabolism.

AEROBIC EXERCISES

These are endurance activities that utilise oxygen for energy production. They are slow, steady-state exercises, which allow time for the systems to supply sufficient oxygen for the oxidation of pyruvic acid. Oxygen supply is maintained throughout and no oxygen debt is incurred. There is therefore no gasping or deep breathing at the end of these activities. Aerobic activities include jogging, walking, swimming, cycling, aerobic classes. (Remember that if the exercises become too fast and vigorous in aerobic classes, the exercise will be anaerobic. Clients should not be short of breath during aerobic activities and should be able to talk or sing whilst exercising.)

ANAEROBIC EXERCISES

These are activities that do not use oxygen for energy production. All activities begin anaerobically and continue until all readily available energy within the muscles is used up; this will last for fifteen to twenty seconds, and is known as the *alactic phase*, as lactic acid is not produced. Further vigorous, fast-moving activities – too fast for the systems to supply oxygen – will result in the breakdown of pyruvic acid into lactic acid. This is known as the *lactic phase*. Lactic acid builds up within the muscle and will eventually inhibit its contraction. Oxygen debt is incurred, which must be repaid at the end of the activity by deep breathing. Anaerobic activities include squash, sprinting, hurdling and fast vigorous actions.

Most sports utilise both energy systems, where the fast vigorous phases are anaerobic and the slower steadier phases are aerobic.

OXYGEN UPTAKE

Oxygen uptake is the amount of oxygen consumed within a certain time: usually one minute. It is known as VO_2. Maximum oxygen uptake is the maximum amount of oxygen taken in and utilised by the muscles to produce energy. The amount of oxygen consumed at rest is around 0.2–0.3 litres per minute, but this increases considerably during exercise, to a point where the system is unable to meet further demand. This point is an individual's *aerobic capacity* or *VO_2 maximum.*

VO_2 maximum can be measured and is used to assess a person's aerobic power or fitness. With training, fitness develops, the heart pumps out more blood, the lungs improve and ventilation increases, with more oxygen taken in. This in turn is delivered to the muscles and used more efficiently. As fitness increases the amount of oxygen taken in increases. Trained athletes have far higher VO_2 maxima than untrained individuals.

Regular training increases the capacity for oxygen uptake and the ability to exercise aerobically for longer periods.

OXYGEN DEBT

As previously explained, during vigorous muscular activity, oxygen cannot be supplied fast enough to the muscle fibres and oxygen supplies are depleted. Energy is therefore generated from the anaerobic breakdown of pyruvic acid, which produces lactic acid. A large percentage of the lactic acid is transported from the muscle to the liver, where it is converted back to glucose or glycogen, but some lactic acid remains in the muscle. After exercise has stopped, extra oxygen is required to metabolise the lactic acid, and to replenish ATP, phosphocreatine and glycogen, as well as increasing the supply of oxygen to the blood and lungs in order to restore the body systems to their normal state. The increase of lactic acid in the blood stimulates the respiratory system, so that breathing increases in depth and rate and oxygen debt is repaid. Lactic acid remaining in the muscle inhibits muscle contraction, producing fatigue.

MUSCLE FATIGUE

Muscle fatigue is the inability of a muscle to sustain a contraction. The contraction becomes progressively weaker and then fails completely as the muscle is unable to produce sufficient energy to meet its needs. Muscle fatigue is thought to be due to depletion of ATP, insufficient glycogen and oxygen and the build-up of lactic acid within a muscle.

QUESTIONS

1 Give three functions of muscle tissue.
2 Name the connective tissue sheath which surrounds a muscle.
3 Name two contractile proteins found in muscle fibres.
4 Complete the following sentence:
Muscle contraction occurs as a result of a stimulus from the ....
5 Explain what happens to a muscle fibre if no cross-bridges remain intact.
6 Name two types of muscle fibre.
7 State which type of muscle fibre depends on aerobic metabolism and which type depends on anaerobic metabolism.
8 Explain what is meant by the term *threshold stimulus*.
9 List any three factors which affect the strength of muscle contraction.
10 Define the following:
   a   tendon
   b   aponeurosis
   c   origin
   d   insertion.

11 Define the term *muscle tone*.
12 Name the structures which transmit information on the degree of tension found in a muscle.
13 Name the chemical which supplies energy for muscle contraction.
14 Briefly explain why energy is supplied by anaerobic metabolism for the first fifteen to twenty seconds of muscular activity.
15 Explain why lactic acid is produced during short, vigorous bursts of activity.
16 Explain the term *oxygen debt*.
17 State what types of exercise and activities utilise aerobic metabolism.
18 Differentiate between aerobic and anaerobic exercises.
19 Explain what is meant by the term VO_2 *maximum*.
20 Define the term *muscle fatigue* and explain how it occurs.

CHAPTER 6

Physical principles relating to exercise

The science or study of body movement is known as kinesiology. As previously explained, movement is normally produced by muscles acting or pulling on bones, resulting in movement at joints. These movements are affected and governed by certain scientific principles. These need to be understood in order to identify muscle work and to devise effective and appropriate exercise schemes.

Force

Any force acting on the body will make it move or affect its movement. When muscles contract they exert a force, which, if strong enough, will produce movement at the joint, for example the biceps muscle must contract with sufficient force to lift the forearm and bend the elbow. The power of the muscle must be great enough to overcome the resistance of any force pulling the other way, in other words the muscle force must be greater than the resisting force for movement to occur.

There are various external forces that can be used to resist movement, such as the pull of gravity or the use of weights, springs, pulley systems, multigyms, etc. Muscles are strengthened when they are made to work against progressively increasing forces.

Certain postural muscles are continually working against the force of gravity to maintain posture. If these muscles relaxed, the body would fall to the ground.

GRAVITY

This is the force that attracts or pulls everything towards the ground. It is a continual pull in a downward direction.

Gravitational pull affects most body movement and must be considered when planning exercises. Movements performed downwards (with gravity) will require different muscle work from those performed upwards (against gravity). Movements in the sagittal and frontal planes are affected by gravity, but movements in the horizontal plane are not. Movements upwards, downwards or sideways will have different relationships with gravity and will require different muscle work. It is therefore very important to consider gravitational pull and to select appropriate starting positions when compiling exercise schemes (see chapter 10).

ANTI-GRAVITY MUSCLES

The upright posture is maintained by particular muscle groups known as postural muscles or anti-gravity muscles. They must work continuously to oppose the pull of gravity and keep the body upright. Any weakness or imbalance of these muscles will affect body alignment and may result in postural deformities.

Regular exercise will maintain muscle strength and balance, thus preventing abnormal postures. If deformities have developed, specific exercises must be practised to stretch the tight muscles and strengthen weak muscles. The anti-gravity muscles are the anterior tibials, the posterior tibials, the quadriceps, the hip extensors, the erector spinae, the abdominals, the trapezius and the rhomboids, the neck extensors and the neck flexors.

THE CENTRE OF GRAVITY

This is an imaginary point at the centre of a body around which it is perfectly balanced. In the standing position the centre of gravity of the human body lies approximately at the second sacral vertebra, but this will vary with the shape and weight distribution of the individual. More weight on the top half raises the centre of gravity, whereas bending the knees or kneeling will lower it.

The lower the centre of gravity the more stable the object will be, so that a person in the lying position is more stable than a person in the standing position.

Stability is an important consideration when planning exercise, as the more stable the body is the easier it is to perform an exercise.

THE LINE OF GRAVITY

This is an imaginary line which falls perpendicularly (vertically) through the centre of gravity. When a person stands upright, the line of gravity passes through the vertex (top of the head), through the mid-cervical vertebrae, in front of the thoracic vertebrae, behind the bodies of the lumbar vertebrae, through the

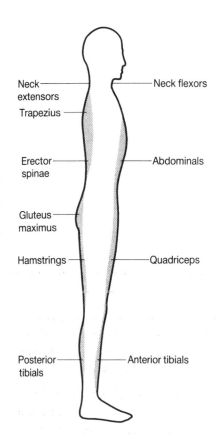

Neck extensors
Trapezius
Erector spinae
Gluteus maximus
Hamstrings
Posterior tibials

Neck flexors
Abdominals
Quadriceps
Anterior tibials

Figure 6.1 *Postural muscles*

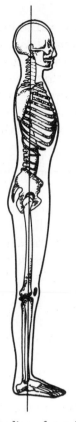

second sacral vertebra, slightly in front of the knee joint and in front of the ankle joint, ending between the ball of the foot and the heel. The line of gravity is a useful measure when examining posture. When the body adopts the correct posture, a line in the same plane but lateral to the line of gravity will fall through the lobe of the ear, the point of the shoulder (the acromion process), the hip joint, to the front of the knee joint (but behind the patella) and in front of the ankle joint, ending between the ball of the foot and the heel (see page 129). The line of gravity will not fall through all these points if posture is incorrect and will move as the position of the body changes.

Figure 6.2 *The line of gravity*

STABILITY

The base of an object is that part that touches the ground. Any object with two or more feet on the ground will have a base that includes the area of the feet and the area of the space in between. The larger the area of the base the greater the stability.

When a person sits on a chair, the base includes the feet of the person and the area between the legs of the chair. When a person is lying down the area of the body surface on the ground is the base. This gives great stability, as it is a large base with a low centre of gravity.

Figure 6.3 *The size of the base in standing, walk standing and stride standing*

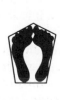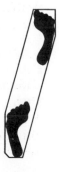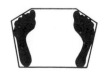

The stability of a body depends on the relationships between the centre of gravity and line of gravity and the base. As has already been mentioned, the lower the centre of gravity, the more stable the body will be. When the line of gravity falls near the centre of the base, the body is stable. As the line of gravity moves towards the edge of the base the body becomes increasingly unstable. If the line of gravity falls outside the base, the body falls over.

When the base is small it is difficult for the line of gravity to remain within it and the body easily falls over, but if the base becomes larger it is easier for the line of gravity to remain within it and the body is more stable. For example, if a person stands with the feet close together, the base is relatively small, being the area of the feet alone. Therefore, if the body moves forward, sideways or backward, the line of gravity will easily fall outside the base and the body will fall over.

However, if a person stands with the feet apart, as in stride standing, the base is much larger, being the area in between the feet as well as the area of the feet. The line of gravity will now stay within the base when the person leans over, and the body will not fall over as it is more stable. Arm and trunk movements are easier to perform when the body is more stable. Whenever the body moves into an unstable position, muscles are immediately brought into play to prevent the body falling over. The smaller the base and the higher the centre of gravity, the greater the muscle power and co-ordination needed to maintain the upright posture and the more difficult it will be to perform exercise. Other factors which increase stability are:

- increased body mass;
- friction between the feet and the ground;
- focusing the vision on a stationary object.

NEWTON'S LAWS OF MOTION

An understanding of these laws is useful when considering exercise, but in-depth study is not required.

Newton's laws state:

1 A body will continue in a state of rest or uniform motion in a straight line unless it is acted on by a force.
2 A change in acceleration of a body is directly proportional to the force and inversely proportional to the mass.
3 To every action there is an equal and opposite reaction.

THE FIRST LAW

The first law explains that a body will remain at rest or continue moving in a straight line unless it is affected by some force. The force may move a stationary object, or may make a moving object move faster or slower or may change the direction of movement. Forces can be applied singly, or many forces can work together in the same direction, or forces can work in opposition to each other.

We can look at examples in everyday life related to muscle work.

- A single force acting on an object will move it in the direction of that force. For example, a man pushing a car will move the car in the direction that he's pushing, providing he pushes hard enough. A muscle pulling on a bone will move the bone, providing the muscle pull is strong enough.

- If two or more forces are acting in the same direction the power or strength of the force will be the sum of the two forces. For example, two people pushing a car in the same direction will move the car in that direction. The strength of the force will be the power of the first person plus the power of the second person and the work will be easier for each of them. In the same way, two muscles pulling together in the same direction will move a bone and the work will be easier for each muscle than if one was working alone. The power will be the sum of the two forces.

- Two forces acting in opposite directions will result in movement in the direction of the greater force. The strength of the force will be the difference between the two forces. For example, two people pushing a car in opposite directions will result in movement in the direction of the one pushing harder. Opposing muscles cannot contract together, because as the prime mover contracts the opposing antagonist always relaxes (this is controlled by nerve impulses and is known as reciprocal relaxation). However, muscles can be made to contract against external forces such as gravity, weights, springs, pulleys or machines. If the muscle force is greater than the external force, movement will occur in the direction of muscle pull. This principle is applied to improve muscle strength. A weight is selected that the muscle is just strong enough to lift, and this weight is lifted a set number of times. As the muscle responds and strengthens a greater weight is used and the procedure is repeated until the required strength is reached. If the muscle power and the weight are equal there will be equilibrium, and therefore no movement. If the weight is greater than the muscle power, movement will occur towards the weight. If the muscle is forced to lift too great a weight the myofibrils may tear, damaging the muscle.

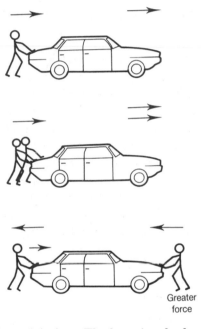

Figure 6.4a, b, c *The forces involved in pushing a car*

Greater force

THE SECOND LAW

The second law explains that an increase in speed will be directly proportional to the force, so that the greater the force, the greater the acceleration. It also depends on the mass: the greater the mass, the lower the acceleration.

For example, if two athletes of equal weight are pushing off from a starting block with equal force, they will accelerate at the same speed. However, if one is much heavier than the other he or she will accelerate more slowly, and will have to use greater force, i.e. muscle power, to produce the same acceleration.

THE THIRD LAW

The third law explains that every action has an equal and opposite reaction. This is important in ball games such as tennis and squash. The harder the ball is hit, the harder it hits the surface and the harder it rebounds. The surface applies a resistance force against the force of the striking ball. The resistance force from hard surfaces is greater than that from softer surfaces, which absorb some of the force. Hard court tennis is faster than grass court tennis, although the standard of play is equal. It is easier to run on hard surfaces than on soft surfaces, as there is a greater opposite reaction propelling one forward. These opposing forces can cause problems for runners, as the constant jarring as the feet hit the ground may cause repetitive stress injuries such as shin splints and spinal problems.

When exercising it is an advantage to work on a sprung floor, which dissipates impact forces and reduces the risk of injury. Well-manufactured training footwear with cushioned soles should be worn to dissipate these forces.

(Some students may require other physical laws and principles related to speed, velocity and so on. These are not within the scope of this book and specialist texts should be referred to.)

Skeletal muscles produce the forces required for mobility. They start and stop movement, they maintain movement, they change the speed of movement, they may accelerate or decelerate actions and they change the direction of movement. Considerably more force is required to start and stop movement and to change direction than to maintain movement in the same direction.

Levers

The principles of leverage also apply to body movement. Levers can be used to make work easier or harder. We are all familiar with the use of a lever to prise the lid off a tin of paint. When a coin is placed under the lid, and a force applied on the other side, the lid lifts up. If the coin does not work, we use a spoon handle or some longer rigid bar, and this will lift the lid because it has greater mechanical advantage.

A lever is a rigid bar which moves around a fixed point called a fulcrum.

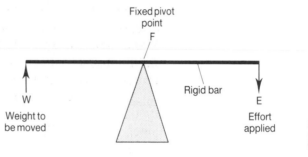

Figure 6.5 *A lever*

A force or effort (E) applied at one point on the lever moves a second force or weight (W) applied at another point.

The distance between the effort and the fulcrum is known as the effort arm (EA) and the distance from the weight to the fulcrum is known as the weight arm (WA).

A lever is balanced when

$$W \times WA = E \times EA$$

If the weight or length of the weight arm increases, the effort or length of the effort arm must also increase. Later we will see how this relates to increasing the work done by muscles.

In the body:

- the rigid bar is the bone;
- the fulcrum is the joint;
- the effort is the pull of the muscle at its point of insertion;
- the weight is the part being moved.

There are three different classes or orders of levers. They are different because of the position of the fulcrum in relation to the effort and the weight.

First order or class (EFW)

In the first order the fulcrum (F) lies between the effort (E) and the weight (W).

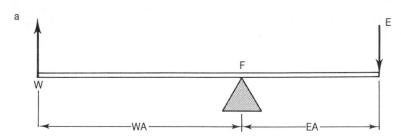

Figure 6.6a *(a) The first order of lever*

Here, the fulcrum may be nearer the weight, giving a longer effort arm, or may lie nearer the effort, giving a longer weight arm. When the effort arm is longer than the weight arm there is mechanical advantage. If the weight arm is longer than the effort arm there is mechanical disadvantage.

We find examples of this first order in everyday life (e.g. a see-saw), but few in the body.

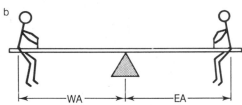

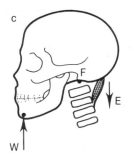

Figure 6.6b, c *(b) Equilibrium on a see-saw*
(c) Extension of the head

If weight × weight arm = effort × effort arm, then the see-saw is balanced, but when one side is greater than the other the see-saw will move down at the end with the greater force. In the human body, during extension of the head the fulcrum lies at the cervical joints. The effort is supplied by the muscle pull at the point of insertion (upper fibres of trapezius) and the weight is the head being moved. In order to move the head backwards, the muscle power and the distance from the fulcrum must be greater than the weight of the head and its distance from the fulcrum.

Second order or class (FWE)

In this order the weight lies between the fulcrum and the effort.

Here, the effort arm will always be longer than the weight arm and consequently there will always be mechanical advantage. This is a lever of power.

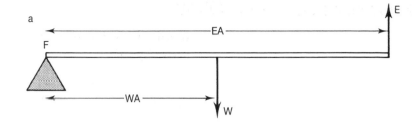

Figure 6.7a, b, c *(a) The second order*
of lever
(b) Lifting a load in a wheelbarrow
(c) Lifting the foot off the ground

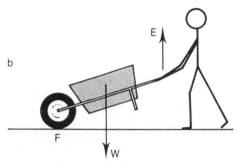

A wheelbarrow has a fulcrum at the wheel, the weight in the middle and the effort at the handle. Because the effort arm is always longer than the weight arm, it is quite easy to lift a heavy load in a wheelbarrow.

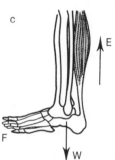

When raising the heel off the ground, the fulcrum is at the metatarso-phalangeal joints, the body weight falls down the leg to the ankle and the effort to lift the heel is from the plantar flexors (gastrocnemius and soleus) at their point of insertion.

THIRD ORDER OF CLASS (FEW)

In this order the effort lies between the fulcrum and the weight.

Here the effort arm will always be shorter than the weight arm and therefore there will be mechanical disadvantage.

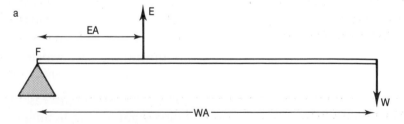

Figure 6.8a *(a) The third order of*
lever

A pair of tongs for picking up objects has the fulcrum at one end, the effort is applied in the middle and the weight lies at the other end.

During flexion of the elbow to lift the forearm, the fulcrum lies at the elbow joint. The effort is applied at the point of insertion of

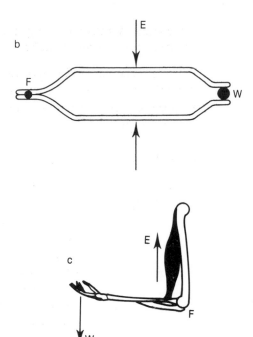

the biceps and brachialis muscles and the weight is the arm being lifted and any weight in the hand.

There are a larger number of third order levers in the body than any other. Although they are levers of mechanical disadvantage, they allow for speed and a wide range of movement.

Figure 6.8b, c *(b) A pair of tongs*
(c) Flexion of the elbow

LEVERAGE RELATED TO MUSCLE WORK

As explained previously, there are examples of all three types of lever to be found in the body, but there are far more of the third class, giving speed and a large range of movement. When power is required we find the second class.

- The *fulcrum* is the joint where movement is taking place.
- The *effort* is provided by the muscle power exerted when the muscle contracts.
- The *effort arm* is the distance from the joint to the point where the muscle inserts (this cannot be changed).
- The *weight* is the part being moved, which can be increased by adding weight to the part.
- The *weight arm* is the distance from the fulcrum to the end of the moving part, which can be increased by adding length, such as a pole or dumb-bell.

Therefore we can increase the effort for the muscle by increasing the weight or lengthening the weight arm.

If muscle power (effort) × effort arm = weight × weight arm, everything is balanced and no movement will occur.

If we increase the muscle power so that muscle power (effort) × effort arm is greater than weight × weight arm, movement will occur.

If we then increase the weight or the length of the weight arm, greater muscle power will be required to product movement.

This principle is used to strengthen muscles. The weight is progressively increased and the muscle is made to lift it a set number of times, with the result that the muscle become stronger (see chapter 8).

EXAMPLES

1 Increasing the work to strengthen abdominal muscles:

Crook lying:
- arms across chest, curl up (short weight arm)
- hands on ears, curl up (longer weight arm)
- arms stretched above head, curl up (longer weight arm)
- arms across chest holding weight, curl up (increased weight)
- arms stretched above head holding weight, curl up (increased weight arm and weight).

This progression continues by increasing the weight to be lifted. Once the muscle can lift the weight ten to fifteen times, the weight can be increased.

2 Increasing the work to strengthen deltoid (Figure 6.9):

Stride standing:
- hand on shoulder, lift arm sideways (short weight arm)
- hand to side, lift arm sideways (longer weight arm)
- hand to side holding pole, lift arm sideways (longer weight arm)
- hand to side holding weight, lift arm sideways (increased weight). This weight can be increased as the muscle gets stronger
- hand to side holding weight at the end of the pole, lift arm sideways (longer weight arm and increased weight).

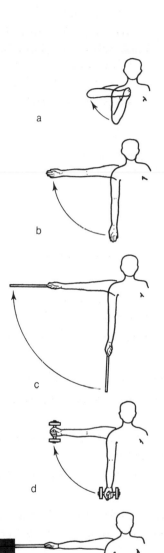

Figure 6.9 *Use of leverage to progress exercise*

T A S K

Show progression for the abductors of the hip joint in the side-lying position using the above five steps.

Q U E S T I O N S

1 Define the terms *gravity* and *centre of gravity*.
2 Where is the approximate position of the centre of gravity in the human body?
3 When assessing posture, list the points through which the line of gravity will fall.
4 Complete the following:
   The base of an object is that part which..................
5 Give any three factors which influence the stability of a body.
6 Explain why it is preferable to exercise on a sprung floor.

7 Draw diagrams to illustrate the three classes of levers.
8 Relate the parts of a lever to the human body.
9 Give two ways in which leverage can be used to increase the resistance to muscle work.
10 Show two ways of using leverage to make the following exercise harder for the gluteus maximus:
   prone lying, raise the leg off the floor, knee bent to right angle.

CHAPTER 7

Muscle work

Muscles work to produce or control movement at joints. When a muscle is working, tension builds up within the muscle and the muscle may shorten, lengthen or remain the same length depending on the action required.

The muscle may be required to move a part, to control the effect of an external force or to hold a specific static position.

Isotonic and isometric work

Muscle work is classified into:

- *Isotonic* – equal tone – the muscle changes in length throughout the movement but the tone remains the same. The muscle may shorten, when the work is known as *concentric* work, or the muscle may lengthen, when the work is known as *eccentric* work. (In practice it is difficult for tone to remain the same throughout the full range of movement because of the difference in the angle of pull across the range. Machines are now able to adjust automatically to keep the tone constant. This work is known as *isokinetic.*)

- *Isometric* – equal length – the length of the muscle does not change, but there is a change in tone. This is also known as static work.

DEFINITIONS

Isotonic work may be concentric or eccentric:

- Concentric work (isotonic shortening) – a muscle working concentrically shortens and thickens, the origin and insertion move towards each other and movement is produced in the joint. For example, in bending the elbow to lift a weight, the elbow flexors shorten to flex the elbow.

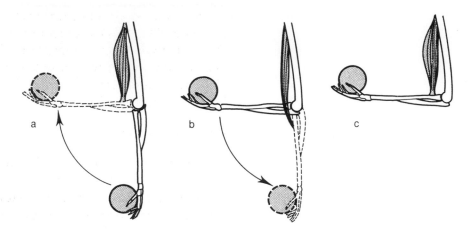

Figure 7.1a, b, c *(a) The biceps working concentrically to lift a ball (b) The biceps working eccentrically to lower a ball (c) The biceps working statically to hold a ball*

- Eccentric work (isotonic lengthening) – a muscle working eccentrically becomes longer and thinner as the origin and insertion move away from each other. The muscle pays out gradually to control the movement produced by some external force such as gravity, springs, etc. For example, when lowering a bucket of water to the ground, the elbow flexors lengthen and pay out gradually to lower the bucket smoothly downwards. If these muscles stopped working the bucket would drop rapidly due to the force of gravity.

Isometric work is also known as static work.

- A muscle working statically does not change in length, but there is an increase in muscle tone. The origin and insertion do not move and there is no joint movement. For example, when holding a bucket of water above the ground, the elbow flexors have to increase in tone to maintain the position, but there is no movement at the elbow joint. Muscles can be made to work statically by pushing against immovable objects or by holding heavy weights or springs.

OTHER EXAMPLES OF CONCENTRIC, ECCENTRIC AND STATIC WORK

CONCENTRIC WORK

Another example of concentric work is standing and raising the arm to the side. This movement of abduction at the shoulder joint is brought about by the contraction of the deltoid. The deltoid becomes shorter and thicker as the insertion moves towards the origin, its power overcomes the pull of gravity and the arm is abducted. The deltoid is working concentrically.

ECCENTRIC WORK

One way to lower the arm would be for all muscles to relax, so that the arm would fall rapidly down to the side. In order to control this movement of adduction, the deltoid now 'pays out' with the insertion moving away from the origin so that the arm is lowered slowly in a controlled manner. The deltoid is working eccentrically.

STATIC WORK

To continue with the same example, the deltoid would work statically if the arm were held out in abduction, allowing no movement. Common static exercises are tightening and holding the gluteal muscles, the abdominals and the quadriceps.

THE USES OF MUSCLE WORK

Concentric muscle work is the most effective for muscle strengthening, although eccentric and static work should also be included.

Eccentric muscle work can sometimes be easier to perform and is useful when re-educating muscles if they cannot perform concentric work. Eccentric work in full and outer range (see below) maintains flexibility but produces muscle soreness.

Static work is easy to perform, but muscle fatigue develops quickly. This is because the constant compression on the blood vessels and capillary networks impedes the blood flow, thus reducing the delivery of oxygen and nutrients and the removal of waste products.

Static work increases the blood pressure and should not therefore be performed by those with heart and blood pressure problems.

Static work should be practised for short periods, with frequent rest intervals. It is also important to perform static holding at different points throughout the muscle range.

Work with a partner.
While one of you performs a movement, the other should try to identify the type of muscle work. For example, standing, swing the right leg out sideways. The abductors are working concentrically.

Range of movement

When muscles contract they move the joint through a certain range.

There are four ranges that a muscle or joint can work through:

1 *Full range* – from full stretch to full contraction, or vice versa.
2 *Outer range* – from full stretch to the mid-point of contraction, or vice versa.
3 *Inner range* – from the mid-point to full contraction, or vice versa.
4 *Middle range* – any distance from the mid-point of the outer range to the mid-point of the inner range, or vice versa.

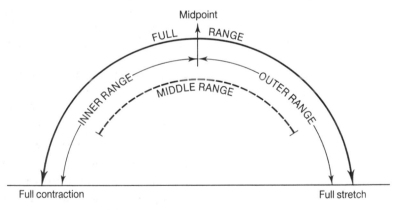

Figure 7.2 *The four ranges of movement*

Full-range work is rarely used for normal activities, but it is essential for maintaining full joint mobility and muscle flexibility and is useful for reducing tension.

Outer-range work is difficult due to the angle of pull of the muscle, and energy is wasted in the compression of joint surfaces (shunting), but exercises in both the full and outer ranges prevent shortening of the muscles and maintain joint mobility. The outer range is used for stretching work.

Inner-range work is used when re-educating weak muscles and for strengthening work as the angle of pull is advantageous, but extreme inner-range work again wastes energy in pulling joint surfaces apart.

The middle range is the range in which muscles are most often used in everyday activities. They are more efficient in this range because the angle of pull of the muscle is nearer 90°, but full joint movement is never achieved in this range.

Remember:

- inner- and middle-range work for re-educating weak muscles and strengthening exercises;
- full-range work for mobilising joints and relieving tension;
- outer-range work for stretching, preventing muscle shortening and maintaining flexibility and end of range movement at joints.

The group action of muscles

When muscles contract to produce movement, they work in groups. Each member of the group has a particular role to play, rather like the members of an orchestra. They work together in a synchronised manner to produce smooth, co-ordinated, efficient movement.

There are four different members, which are named according to their function. They are the agonists or prime movers, the antagonists, the synergists and the fixators:

- The *agonists* or *prime movers* are the muscles that contract to produce the required movement (prime action). For example, abduction of the hip joint is produced by the abductors; therefore the gluteus medius, the gluteus minimus and the tensor fasciae latae are the agonists or prime movers.
- The *antagonists* lie on the opposite side of the joint from the agonists. They are the opposite group, which must relax and lengthen in a controlled manner so that the movement produced by the agonists is performed smoothly. For example, when the abductors are contracting to abduct the hip the opposite group, the adductors, must relax. Therefore the adductors magnus, longus, brevis, pectineus and gracilis are the antagonists.
- The *synergists* assist the prime movers to produce the most efficient movement. They may alter the angle of pull of the prime mover or prevent unwanted movement. For example, during abduction of the hip the deep hip muscles will prevent the hip rotating, so that maximum effort is put into abduction. Therefore the piriformis and the obturator muscles are the synergists.

- The *fixators* ensure that the prime movers act from a fixed base. They stabilise and prevent unnecessary movements in surrounding joints. For example, during abduction of the hip joint the pelvis is held steady. Therefore the trunk side flexors and abductors of the opposite side are the fixators.

The agonists and antagonists are the most vital members of the group and require identification when analysing muscle work. When the agonists are contracting to produce movement, the antagonists must relax to allow the movement to take place. This is known as reciprocal relaxation and can be used as a technique for stretching muscles (see chapter 8). It is sufficient to remember that synergists and fixators are also contributing to the movement, as their identification is frequently difficult.

The muscles acting on a joint are arranged around the joint. Some are superficial while others are deep. The agonists and antagonists are arranged as opposite pairs – flexors opposite extensors, abductors opposite adductors, medial rotators opposite lateral rotators. When the flexors are the agonists, the extensors will be the antagonists and vice versa. Other smaller muscles will be the synergists and fixators. The patterns of movement are synchronised in the motor cortex and the appropriate impulses are conveyed to the muscles via their motor nerves.

The balance between agonists and antagonists is very important, as tightness and shortening or over-stretching and weakness of one group will affect the function of the other. A muscle imbalance will be produced, resulting in stresses on the underlying joints and ligaments. These stresses may result in deformity and pain. Exercises must always be planned to maintain a balance between agonists and antagonists.

Analysis of muscle work

All exercise schemes require careful planning to ensure that the set objectives are realised. For corrective schemes, the exercises must be carefully planned to target specific muscles or groups: some will require strengthening, while others will require stretching. For general schemes, all the main muscle groups must be included and balance maintained between opposing muscles.

Planning exercise schemes therefore requires the ability to analyse muscle work. First of all, the starting position must be considered, as this determines the effect of gravity on the movement. This is followed by identification of the moving joint, the direction of movement and the muscles producing that movement. Then we consider the type of muscle work and the range of movement. To analyse muscle work, therefore, we must follow this procedure:

1 Give the starting position.
2 Name the moving joint, e.g. hip, shoulder, etc.
3 Name the direction of movement, e.g. flexion, abduction, etc.
4 Name the prime movers, i.e. the muscles producing the movement.
5 Name the type of muscle work, i.e. concentric, eccentric or static.
6 Name the range of movement, i.e. inner, outer, middle or full.

The type of muscle work poses the most difficult problem to most students. Remember:

- If the muscle is shortening and the origin and insertion are moving nearer to each other, the work is concentric.

- If the movement is produced by an external force such as gravity, weights or springs and the muscle is lengthening and paying out to control the movement, so that the origin and insertion are moving away from each other, the work is eccentric.

- If the muscle is contracting but producing no movement at the joint, the work is static.

Exercises performed in different starting positions will have different muscle work, for example abduction and adduction of the hip joint performed in different positions, as shown below.

Position:	lying supine
Movement:	part legs
Moving joint:	hip
Direction of movement:	abduction
Prime movers:	the abductors (gluteus medius, minimus and tensor fasciae latae)

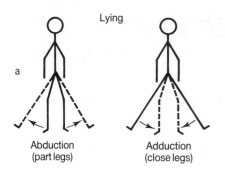

Figure 7.3 *Abduction and adduction of the legs (a) lying (b) side lying (c) lying with legs against a wall*

Muscle work:	concentric (muscle shortens producing the movement)
Range:	inner
Movement:	close legs
Moving joint:	hip
Direction of movement:	adduction
Prime movers:	adductors (adductors longus, magnus, brevis, pectineus, gracilis)
Muscle work:	concentric
Range:	outer

When the legs are opened and closed in the lying position gravity does not affect the movement, since gravitational pull is downwards and this movement is in the horizontal plane.

Both the abductors and adductors work concentrically.

Now if we change the starting position but do the same movement the muscle work changes.

Position:	lying on side
Movement:	upper leg raise
Moving joint:	hip joint
Direction of movement	abduction
Prime movers:	abductors (as before)
Muscle work:	concentric (muscle shortens)
Range:	inner

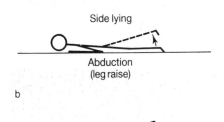

(This movement is against the pull of gravity.)

Movement:	lowering leg
Moving joint:	hip joint
Direction of movement:	adduction
Prime movers:	abductors (because gravity will pull the leg down)
Muscle work:	eccentric
Range:	inner

Gravity pulls the leg down, therefore the adductors do not need to work, but the abductors work eccentrically to prevent the leg from falling.

Thus in this starting position the muscle work changes: only the abductors work, first concentrically and then eccentrically to produce controlled movement and counteract the pull of gravity.

If we change the starting position yet again, the muscle work will change again.

Lying legs against a wall

c

Abduction
(part legs)

Adduction
(close legs)

Position:	lying with legs at right angles to trunk
Movement:	part legs
Moving joint:	hip joint
Direction of movement:	abduction
Prime movers:	adductors (because gravity will pull the legs out)
Muscle work:	eccentric
Range:	outer

Movement:	close legs
Moving joint:	hip joint
Direction of movement:	adduction
Prime movers:	adductors
Muscle work:	concentric
Range:	outer

Only the adductors work in this position, first eccentrically to produce controlled movement and counteract the pull of gravity. They then work concentrically to draw the legs in.

T A S K

Work out the muscle work of elbow flexion and extension in the following starting positions.
(Remember that the biceps flexes the elbow and the triceps extends the elbow.)

a stride standing (arms at side) – raise hand to touch shoulder

b as above – lower hand back down

c yard stride standing – bring hand in to touch shoulder

d as above – bring hand back out to yard

e head rest stride standing – raise hand up to elevation

f as above – lower hand back to head.

The classification of movement

Movements may be classified as shown in Figure 7.4.

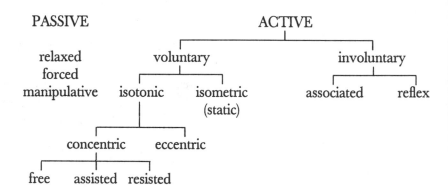

Figure 7.4 *The classification of movement*

PASSIVE MOVEMENTS

These movements are performed by an external force, and the client's own muscles are inactive, i.e. do not contract. The therapist moves the joint, but the client plays no active part. These movements are used to maintain or increase the mobility in joints.

They may be classified as:

- relaxed passive movements – performed within the existing range;
- forced passive movements – performed beyond the existing range;
- manipulative passive movements – these are forced movements performed under anaesthetic and are carried out to break down adhesions that are limiting joint movement.

Passive movements should be carried out under medical supervision only.

ACTIVE MOVEMENTS

These may be voluntary, i.e. under the control of the will, or involuntary, i.e. not under the control of the will.

INVOLUNTARY MOVEMENTS

These are not controlled by the will and may be:

- *reflex* movements, such as blinking or movement away from hot or painful conditions;
- *associated* movements, which are made by the fixators and synergists during active movements.

VOLUNTARY MOVEMENTS

These movements are controlled by the will and are the result of the voluntary action of muscles. They may be:

- *isometric* (static), where the muscles do not change in length but increase in tone and no movement is produced at the joint;
- *isotonic*, where the muscles change in length and produce movement at the joints. Isotonic movements may be concentric (muscle shortening) or eccentric (muscle lengthening).

Concentric movements may be further subdivided into assisted, free and resisted:

- *Assisted active exercise* – when muscle power is inadequate to produce a desired movement, its power can be helped by the use of an external force acting with the muscle pull. The movement is thus assisted.
- *Free active exercise* is movement where the working muscles are subjected only to the forces of gravity acting upon the part being moved.
- *Resisted active exercise* is movement where the action of the muscles is resisted by an external force, e.g. weights, springs, etc. This resistance acts against the muscle pull. It can be increased progressively to develop muscle power and endurance.

QUESTIONS

1 Name the two main types of muscle work.
2 Define the terms *concentric work* and *eccentric work* and give one example of each.
3 Explain the four ranges of movement.
4 Name each member which contributes to the group action of muscles.
5 Define the terms:
  a prime mover (agonist)
  b antagonist.
6 List the points to consider when analysing muscle work.

7 Analyse the muscle work of the following actions carried out in stride-standing position:
  a raise the arm out to the side to shoulder level
  b lower the arm back to the side.
  Now analyse these movements when the body is lying supine.
8 Define the terms *active movement* and *passive movement*.

The components of fitness

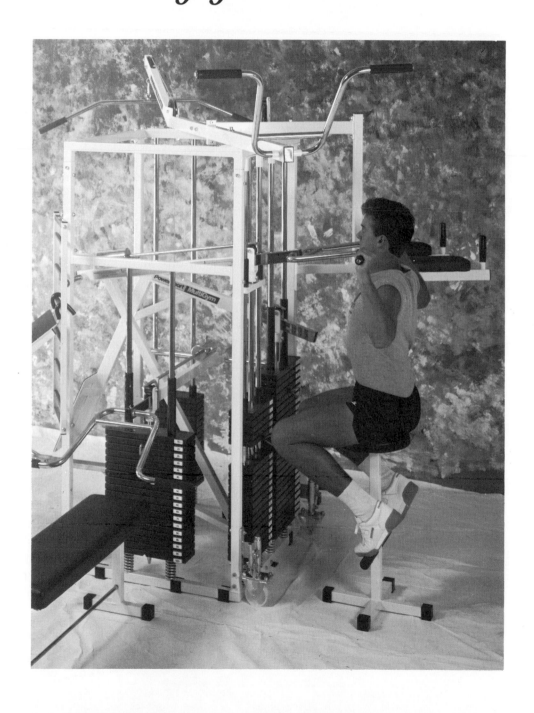

Introduction

'Fitness' means having sufficient energy and skill to cope in one's environment. Fitness is specific to the individual and ranges from the optimum fitness required by top athletes through to the lowest level required barely to cope with daily tasks.

Fitness and health are interrelated, but it is important to distinguish between the two. Health may be defined as 'freedom from disease' or 'a state of physical, mental and social well-being'; it is therefore possible to be healthy (free from disease) but unfit. It is also possible to be superbly fit and compete at the highest level while suffering ill health. Many top athletes continue competing or training when suffering from colds, infections, and so on.

Improving a person's fitness means improving the physiological functioning of the various body systems, which in turn will improve his or her capacity to function and, thus, quality of life. Improvement is brought about by overloading the systems, in other words by making demands on them over and above those required by normal activities, and continuing progressively to work them harder.

Overload should always be appropriate to the fitness level of the individual. It must be of sufficient intensity, frequency and duration to stress the systems, but must be increased gradually. Too much overload too rapidly applied can over-stress and damage the systems. A fitness programme must be specific to the individual and must consider the desired outcome. It must be carefully structured to increase fitness in a consistent and progressive manner. Before embarking on a fitness programme two questions should be asked:

1 What is the desired outcome?
2 What is the current fitness level (the starting point)?

The strategy is then planned from this starting point.

CHAPTER 8

The components of fitness

General fitness programmes must be structured to stress all the systems that contribute to fitness. The physical components of fitness are recognised as:

- Cardio-respiratory endurance (aerobic endurance)
- Muscle strength and endurance
- Flexibility
- Body composition.

In addition to these physical components, one must include:

- speed;
- skill (including co-ordination, balance, timing, rhythm, agility).

Total fitness must also give consideration to:

- nutrition (i.e. diet);
- rest and relaxation.

Athletes, sport and fitness enthusiasts and dancers require a basic level of fitness and, in addition, require skills specific to their sport. They must carry out specific training tasks to meet the demands of their particular sport or activities, placing greater emphasis on some components than others. For example, marathon runners need to improve long-term aerobic energy systems, cyclists require muscle strength in the legs, shot putters and javelin throwers require muscle strength in the shoulder and arm, and so on. However, it is important to keep a balance between the components and to guard against over-development of one at the expense of another. If training ceases, the effects of training will regress and fitness levels will return to pre-training levels. The effects of training over a long period will remain for a longer period after training stops. The effects of short-duration training regress more quickly.

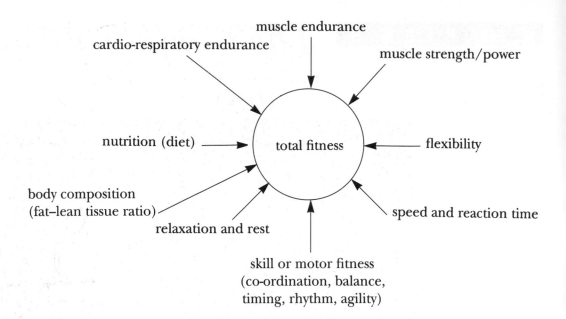

Figure 8.1 *Input necessary for fitness*

Cardio-respiratory endurance

Cardio-vascular, cardio-pulmonary and aerobic endurance are other terms used for this aspect of fitness. They all refer to the efficiency of the heart, circulation and lungs at taking in oxygen, transporting it and transferring it to muscle tissue.

Before exercise, the body is in a balanced state known as homeostasis, where the systems meet the body's metabolic needs. When exercise begins, the systems must respond rapidly to the increased demand for nutrients and oxygen to produce ATP. Cardiac output must increase, and therefore heart rate and stroke volume rise. More air must be taken in by the lungs, so breathing becomes faster and deeper. Haemoglobin levels rise in order to transport more oxygen to the muscle cells, where it will metabolise glycogen and fatty acids for energy. The mitochondria within the cells increase in size and number and the oxygen is utilised more efficiently.

The exercise must continue at a steady state or pace, so that the oxygen supply can meet the demand, for aerobic work. If the exercise becomes too fast and vigorous, the systems will be unable to supply oxygen fast enough to meet the demand and the work will become anaerobic. The capacity of the body to work aerobically will increase with training.

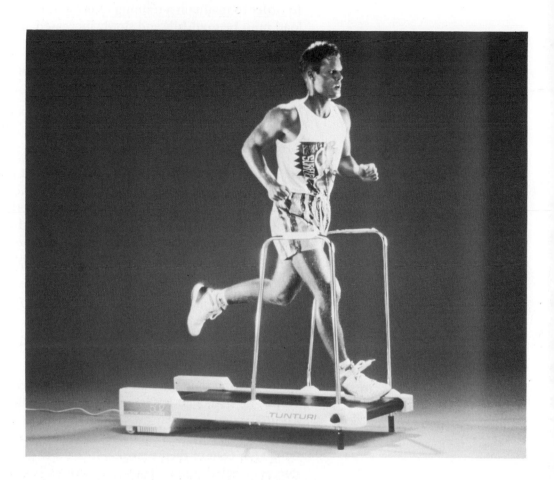

Figure 8.2 *One of many types of aerobic activity*

The heart rate will be progressively lowered for the same workload, indicating greater efficiency. The aerobic capacity VO_2max will increase with training. Average aerobic capacity is around 40–45 ml/kg, but well-trained endurance athletes may have a VO_2max of 60–70 ml/kg (see page 65).

METHODS OF IMPROVING CARDIO-RESPIRATORY ENDURANCE

Cardio-respiratory endurance will improve in response to regular aerobic activities such as:

- jogging;
- swimming;
- walking;

- cross-country skiing;
- cycling;
- aerobic dance or exercise programmes.

In order to maintain a training effect and improve fitness the work load must be gradually and slowly increased. There are three variables to consider:

- the intensity of the exercise – how hard it is;
- the duration of exercise – how long it lasts;
- the frequency of exercise – how often it is performed.

INTENSITY

Heart rate increases with exercise, therefore it is an excellent indicator of how hard the body is working. The rate varies considerably between different people and in the same person under different conditions. The heart rate is the same as the pulse rate and can be taken at pulse points throughout the body. The usual point for reading pulse rate is at the wrist (the radial pulse point).

- The average male resting pulse is between 72–76 beats per minute.
- The average female resting pulse is between 76–80 beats per minute.

These are **average** values and considerable variations will be found. Fit people **have** a far lower resting pulse rate than the unfit. **Endurance** athletes may have pulse rates as low as 30–40 beats per minute. Healthy adults should exercise at a target heart rate of 60–90 per cent of their maximal heart rate depending on their current level of fitness. Those who are unfit should exercise at the lower end while those who are already quite fit should exercise at the higher end of their target range.

To obtain an estimate of maximum heart rate (MHR) deduct the client's age from 220. For example, for a 40-year-old, maximum heart rate will be $220 - 40 = 180$ beats per minute.

The pulse rate must not exceed this MHR during aerobic exercise, as it will produce too much stress. Initially, for endurance training, exercise should be done at 60 per cent of MHR. For a 40-year-old this will be:

$$180 \times \frac{60}{100} = 108 \text{ beats/min. (this is the target heart rate or training rate.)}$$

The client should exercise with sufficient intensity to maintain this pulse rate for fifteen to thirty minutes duration. After four to six weeks it will be safe to exercise at 70 per cent of maximum heart rate;

$$180 \times \frac{70}{100} = 126 \text{ beats/min.}$$

Eventually, this will build up to 80–85 per cent of MHR.

Therefore, for this client

Age	MHR	Target Zone
40	180	108–153

DURATION

This is the actual time that a person is exercising at the target heart rate. It does not include the warm-up and cool-down periods. This part of an exercise programme will last for fifteen to thirty minutes. Initially, after a warm-up and stretch of fifteen to twenty minutes, the client will perform a fifteen-minute programme, maintaining the target heart rate, and then cool down. This time will gradually increase to 30 minutes as fitness improves.

FREQUENCY

This is the number of sessions per week, which may be two to three times a week for an unfit beginner, moving up to three to four times per week as fitness improves.

PLANNING THE TRAINING PROGRAMME

Any one of these three variables, or any combination of them, must increase as fitness develops, in order to maintain the effects of training. The aerobic activity that provides the greatest enjoyment is usually the most successful, as motivation is greater.

All athletes require a basic level of cardio-vascular endurance and frequently combine running with other specific training. Continuous training involving low effort over a period of time, where breathing is easy, will improve the aerobic systems.

Interval training, where high effort is followed by recovery intervals, will improve both aerobic and anaerobic systems. This is a more effective way of improving overall fitness. Various forms of running are used, in combination with weight training and circuit training:

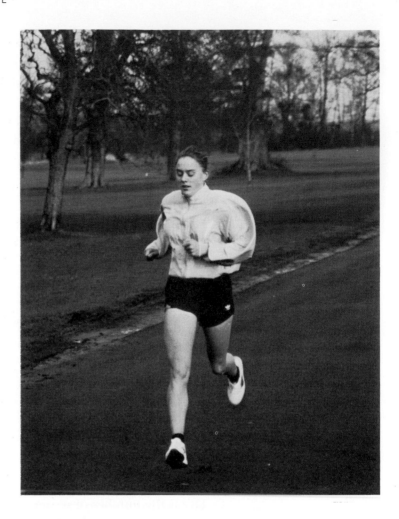

Figure 8.3 *Running*

- *Long continuous running or slow distance running.* This uses low-level effort over a long period of time. Initially, this involves jogging at the target heart rate (60–80 per cent of MHR) for a certain distance in a set period of time (this dictates the pace). Next, the distance is maintained but the time is reduced, or the time maintained but the distance increased, in order to achieve a faster pace. This develops aerobic endurance, and trains the body to use fatty acids as fuel, but it does not develop speed or power.

- *Varied-pace running* (Swedish Fartlek). This varies the pace at specific intervals throughout the run. Continuous steady-pace running is interrupted at intervals by quick sprints. This will combine both anaerobic and aerobic energy systems and is a more realistic training for most sports. It can be varied to use only aerobic systems if low effort is used in all stages.

It may involve running over different terrain, through forests and fields, uphill and downhill, on sand, gravel and grass.

Tracks are very carefully graded for their degree of difficulty. A programme may include:

1 ten to fifteen minutes' jogging;

2 five minutes' rapid walk;

3 one mile slow distance running;

4 ten minutes' rapid walk;

5 five sprints interspersed with jogging over 100 metres.

- *Interval training.* This involves fast training interspersed with slow work, performed in a certain amount of time or over a measured distance. The slow or light work period allows the oxygen debt incurred during the fast work to be repaid. This method will improve both aerobic and anaerobic systems.

- *Pick-up sprint training.* This increases the speed of work. It begins with walking, moving on to jogging, then striding and sprinting, and ending up with walking again. The process is repeated as often as possible. This improves both aerobic and anaerobic systems and trains athletes to pick up speed quickly.

- *Cross-training.* Many athletes believe in and derive benefit from cross-training. This combines different forms of training. For example, cycling may be combined with swimming: the swimming will not improve cycling prowess, but it will maintain endurance qualities while allowing the recovery of the cycling muscles. It is also more interesting and motivating to add variety rather than keep to one training mode.

THE EFFECTS OF ENDURANCE TRAINING

- The heart increases in size and volume.

- The efficiency of the heart improves: it pumps out a larger volume of blood per beat (stroke volume) and therefore a larger quantity per minute (known as cardiac output).

- The heart rate decreases: the heart rests for a longer period, which reduces effort.

- There is an increase in the size and number of blood vessels in the heart and skeletal muscle.

- There is an increase in the density of capillaries in the heart and skeletal muscle, and therefore an improvement in the delivery of oxygen and the removal of waste.

- There is an increase in the size and number of mitochondria, which enables oxygen to be used more efficiently.

- There is an increase in glycogen stores and glycolytic enzymes.

- The aerobic capacity (VO_2max) is increased.

- The anaerobic threshold is raised, so that aerobic metabolism is used for longer periods, increasing the capacity to exercise without fatigue.
- The rate and depth of respiration increases, improving ventilation.
- Fats are utilised for energy production, which reduces body fat.
- Bones are strengthened in response to the stresses placed on them.

DANGERS

- Repetitive stress injuries, mainly of the ankles, knees and back, and shin splint injuries
- Dehydration.

PRECAUTIONS

- Build up the training gradually. Do not exceed maximum heart rate (MHR). Begin at 60 per cent of MHR, working up to 80 per cent as fitness develops.
- Do not exercise if there is any pain present in musculoskeletal structures.
- Do not exercise if suffering from colds, fevers, flu, etc.
- Stop exercising if pain develops.
- Drink fluid after the training session or during long-distance running to prevent dehydration.
- Wear well-fitting, well-cushioned, appropriate footwear.
- Wear loose, absorbent clothing.

Muscle fitness

Muscles respond to overload training in different ways, depending on the type of training:

- Muscle strength will increase in response to progressive overload over a period of time. Strength develops through high resistance with low repetitions.
- Muscle bulk will increase with strength, but one or two lifts at maximal resistance must be performed to improve bulking.
- Muscle endurance will increase in response to low resistance with high repetitions.
- Muscle power and explosive power will increase in response to plyometric training, involving muscle contraction following a rapid stretch.

MUSCLE STRENGTH

This refers to the maximal force a muscle can develop against resistance. It is measured by the maximum weight that can be lifted in a single effort. This is known as one repetition maximum (1RM). It is established by trial and error, using increasingly heavy weights, until the maximum is reached, for example by performing one lift of 10 kg, one of 12 kg and one at 14 kg, etc., until the maximum weight that can be lifted is reached.

Overloading a muscle with a weight of two-thirds of the muscle's maximum load over a period of time will increase strength and bulk.

Initially, an increase in strength is the result of the recruitment of more motor units. Each motor unit stimulates a large number of muscle fibres to contract. Therefore, the more motor units recruited, the more fibres will be contracting, which will increase strength. Further strength develops as a result of an increase in the contractile proteins (myosin and actin) and in the size and number of myofibrils. These factors also increase muscle bulk.

Males bulk more readily than females, due to higher levels of the male hormone testosterone, which is necessary for the synthesis of actin and myosin. However, females will develop strength in response to progressive weight training. Larger stores of ATP, PC and enzymes required for quick energy are found in muscle fibres as a result of strength training.

METHODS OF STRENGTHENING

Resistance may be applied in many ways, but some of these methods are not measurable, and so accurate progression is not possible. Muscles can be made to work against:

- one's own body weight, e.g. press-ups (these are known as callisthenics) – not measurable;
- the resistance provided by a partner, e.g. pushing or pulling against a partner – not measurable;
- free weights, e.g. sand bags, weight boots, ankle and wrist weights, dumb-bells and bar bells;
- springs and pulleys;
- specialised equipment, such as rowing machines, exercise bikes, multigyms and other forms of resistance machines;
- water – not measurable.

Resistance may be applied to isometric or isotonic muscle work.

ISOMETRIC WORK

Isometric work is also called static work: tension develops in the muscle, but the muscle does not change in length. Resistance can be applied to isometric work by pushing against immovable objects such as the wall, table, floor, etc., and allowing no movement.

The best results are obtained if the muscle is worked at different points throughout the range, for example performing two to five contractions at the end of the inner range, the beginning and end of the middle range and the end of the outer range, where each contraction lasts around five seconds.

The disadvantages of isometric resistance work are:

- There is no alternate contraction and relaxation of the muscle, and therefore no pumping action to deliver blood. The pressure maintained on the capillary networks in the muscles prevents the delivery of nutrients and oxygen and fatigue quickly develops.
- There is an increase in blood pressure; isometric work should not be performed by the elderly or by anyone with heart or blood pressure problems.
- Strength can be developed through isometric work, but it is impossible to measure accurate progression.
- Strength may not be developed through the entire range.

ISOTONIC WORK

Resistance may be applied to concentric work (muscle shortening) and to eccentric work (muscle lengthening), and is usually applied to both. Resistance is applied to concentric work as the muscle contracts to lift the weight, and to eccentric work as the part is lowered back to the starting position. The concentric phase can be referred to as the positive phase, and the eccentric phase as the negative phase. For example, biceps curl is concentric work for biceps, while lowering back to the starting position is eccentric work for the biceps. The force and tension developed in the muscle will vary across the range because as the bones move so the angle of pull alters. The force is greatest at the beginning to initiate the movement.

ISOKINETIC WORK

Special machines have been developed for this type of work. Isokinetic muscle work maintains maximal tension across the full range of movement. Resistance to this type of muscle work is provided by special machines, which automatically adapt the resistance as the muscle contracts, so that tension is constant throughout the range.

Techniques of strength training

Exercise schemes may be required either for general body strengthening or for the strengthening of specific muscles or groups, or for both. When strengthening muscles it is important to maintain a balance between opposing muscles, i.e. the agonists and antagonists.

In order to maintain the training effect and increase strength the overload principle must apply. The work must be gradually increased, considering the three variables:

- intensity – how much weight;
- duration – how many repetitions;
- frequency – how often the work is performed.

PLANNING STRENGTHENING PROGRAMMES

- Assess goals – to what end is improvement required?
- Assess the present level of strength – which muscles require strengthening?
- Set the objectives.
- Plan the warm-up.
- Plan the stretch routine.
- Plan general strengthening exercises.
- Plan specific strengthening exercises, selecting the resistance carefully to suit the strength level.
- Plan the cool-down and include some stretching.

GENERAL STRENGTH TRAINING

These schemes include strengthening exercises for all the large muscle groups of the legs, trunk and arms. General schemes may include exercises against gravity, against one's own body weight, against resistance from a partner, or using weights such as dumb-bells, poles, ankle and wrist weights, medicine balls and so on. They may be performed individually or as a class. Exercise classes generally include some strengthening work.

Circuits may be constructed, where each station (area) provides an exercise for one part of the body. These are organised in a circle around the room. Six to ten exercises are carefully planned so that the client can progress easily from one to the next, using different muscles at each station. Care must be taken to explain each movement before commencing the circuit, and each exercise should be practised to ensure accuracy. The number of repetitions of each exercise and the load will depend upon the level of fitness

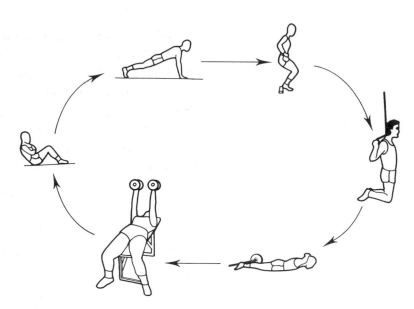

Figure 8.4 *Circuit training*

of the individual and can be increased as strength develops. Some circuits offer weights interspersed with an aerobic activity such as jogging or cycling. This is an excellent way of improving strength and endurance.

SPECIFIC STRENGTH TRAINING

These schemes are designed to improve the strength and bulk of specific muscles, such as the biceps, quadriceps or deltoid, using weight training. In order to increase strength the weight lifted must be over two-thirds of the maximum possible weight (i.e. over 66 per cent of 1RM).

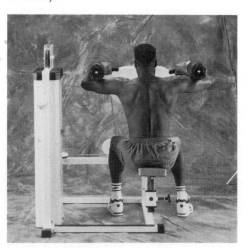

Figure 8.5 *Use of resistance to improve muscle strength*

It is very important to keep an accurate record of the programme and progress. Bulk is measured using a tape measure, while strength is gauged by the maximum weight that can be lifted in a single lift (1RM). Data are recorded as follows:

- bulk – measure around the widest point, always measuring at the same point when the muscle is contracted (see chapter 10);
- the weight lifted – this should be 66 per cent or more of the maximum possible weight;
- the set – the number of times the weight is lifted without a rest (between six and ten lifts);
- the number of sets performed (between one and five sets, allowing a one-minute rest period between sets).

As strength develops it is usual to increase the number of repetitions in one set gradually from six to ten, and to build up from one to three sets. This is recorded as follows:

- 10 kg lifted six times (i.e. one set): 10 kg $\times$ 6 $\times$ 1;
- 10 kg lifted in two sets of six: 10 kg $\times$ 6 $\times$ 2.

Opinions vary as to the effectiveness of different numbers of repetitions: some favour two to six lifts, while others favour ten lifts. In either case, the weight lifted is at least 66 per cent of the maximum for that number of lifts. Each set is repeated three times. Those requiring strength tend to use six to ten lifts, while those developing bulk tend to use a maximum of two to six lifts with maximum weight. It is recommended that strength training is practised three times per week. This allows the muscles and tissues time to recover.

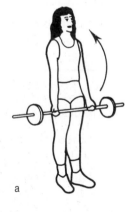
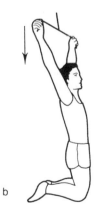

Figure 8.6 *(a) Weight training for the biceps*
(b) Weight training for the latissimus dorsi

a

b

THE PYRAMID METHOD

This is effective for strength, bulk and endurance. As the weight increases the repetitions decrease. For example, a client might perform five repetitions at 2 kg, four at 3 kg, three at 4 kg and two at 5 kg, and then reverse the order, reducing the weight and increasing the repetitions. The maximum weight that can be lifted twice is assessed, and the pyramid is constructed from that starting point. A one-sided regime is sometimes used, working up to maximum weight and then resting.

PRECAUTIONS

- Set realistic objectives.
- Select weights appropriate to the individual's strength level.
- Check the weights for safety.
- Start with an easy programme, with light weights and few lifts.
- Choose a good stable starting position.
- Secure the weights so that they cannot move or slide.
- Maintain a good body alignment.
- Perform the lift carefully and slowly for maximum effect (momentum plays a part in fast movement and can result in trauma).
- The rest between each lift should be at least one or two seconds. Allow one minute's recovery time between sets.
- Increase the number of lifts up to 30 (10×3) and then increase the weight.
- Do not hold the breath when lifting, as this can cause an increase in blood pressure and increases the load on the heart. Holding the breath can also increase intra-abdominal pressure, which can cause hernia.
- Exhale as you lift, inhale as you lower.
- Work different muscle groups. Change the exercises so that different muscles are stressed. Allow time for recovery.
- Maintain a balance between agonist and antagonist.
- Replace weights and all apparatus neatly and safely.

THE EFFECTS OF STRENGTH TRAINING

The physiological effects of muscle strengthening are:

- the recruitment of more motor units, which increases the strength of the contraction;
- a faster neuro-muscular response, which increases the speed of contraction;
- an increase in the size and number of myofibrils, which increases strength and bulk;
- an increase in the contractile proteins myosin and actin;
- an increase in glycogen stores;
- an increase in blood flow to the muscles due to dilation (although there is no increase in the number of blood vessels or capillary networks as with endurance training).

THE DANGERS OF STRENGTH TRAINING

The dangers of strength training are:

- muscle strain and even rupture of fibres if too much overload is applied;
- muscle fatigue and soreness if repetitions are too high and rest periods are too short;
- trauma if weights are not properly secure so that they fall and cause damage;
- damage to the moving joints and their connective tissue components if the positioning of the joint is incorrect or if the lifts are casually performed;
- over-stress of other joints through poor posture and poor technique.

T A S K

Work with a partner. One person should sit in a high sitting position, with thighs supported and feet off the floor. Assess 3RM for the quadriceps muscle. (This is the maximum weight that can be lifted three times.) Strap increasing weights around the ankle until the appropriate weight is reached. The foot should be dorsi-flexed, and the knee must straighten maximally and lock.

MUSCLE ENDURANCE

This is the ability of the muscles to perform repeated contractions continuously over a period of time. The main difference in training for endurance as opposed to training for strength is that lighter weights are used and the repetitions are increased. The method employed is the same.

For endurance, the weight is kept below 66 per cent of the maximum and repeated 25–50 times or more. Training must be repeated three to five times per week. Speed can be improved using high-speed contractions with low resistance. To increase power (speed × strength), three sets of fifteen high-speed contractions with 30–60 per cent of maximal load should be performed.

Explosive power will improve using *plyometrics*. These are jumping, leaping and hopping movements, where the prime mover is stretched before contraction. The speed of the stretch is an important factor. When a muscle is stretched, the stretch receptors within the muscle are stimulated. This increases the strength of the following contraction. The longer and faster the stretch, the greater the following concentric contraction. There is a danger of damaging joints and producing micro-tears in muscle fibres when performing these exercises. They must only be performed by the very fit and only after adequate warm-up.

THE EFFECTS OF MUSCLE ENDURANCE TRAINING

The physiological effects of training for endurance are:

- an increase in the number and size of blood vessels in the muscles;
- an increase in the number of capillary networks;
- an increase in the number of mitochondria in the muscle cells;
- an increase in the number of oxidative enzymes, which extract oxygen from the blood; the aerobic capacity of the muscles is therefore improved;
- an increase in glycogen stores and glycolitic enzymes used for energy.

Flexibility or suppleness

This refers to the range of movement possible at a joint or group of joints. A joint will move through an arc of movement from one point to another, for example from full flexion to full extension. (See chapter 7.)

Joints must be considered separately, as flexibility is specific to each joint. However, an activity such as throwing a ball will require flexibility at more than one joint, and therefore the movement at all of those joints must be considered. Flexibility can be increased through regular training and will contribute to efficient technique, improved performance and the prevention of injury. There are a number of factors that influence flexibility:

- Joint structure
- Age
- Training
- Sex
- Body temperature
- Strength training.

JOINT STRUCTURE

This is the main factor influencing flexibility. It includes:

- the shape and contour of the articulating surfaces (the tighter the fit the more limited the range);

- the tension of the connective tissue components (i.e. the capsule and supporting ligaments);
- the tension of the muscles and tendons acting on and surrounding the joint, which is governed by the stretch reflex (where there is muscle imbalance, flexibility will be limited by the tight muscles).

AGE

Generally, ageing reduces flexibility, but training and activity will influence the degree of loss. Young children are very flexible and, depending on the level of activity, this flexibility continues to increase up to adolescence at around fifteen years of age. After the age of fifteen there is a natural decrease in flexibility. The rate of decrease will depend upon the training, exercise and activities practised by the individual. Research indicates that flexibility can be increased for all age groups if appropriate exercises are undertaken, but the rate of increase will be greater in younger age groups and will decline with age.

TRAINING

As stated above, training and the selection of appropriate exercise will increase flexibility for all age groups. Those individuals, such as gymnasts and ballet dancers, who continue with uninterrupted training programmes will have greater flexibility than the untrained.

SEX

It has been suggested that females are more flexible than males, although the evidence is inconclusive. Females on the whole have lighter and smaller bones, which may influence flexibility. In the main they have a shorter leg length and lower centre of gravity, making certain movements easier. They are also designed for flexibility of the pelvic region to facilitate childbirth.

BODY TEMPERATURE

The elevation of body temperature increases flexibility. Therefore, warm-up exercises must be performed before flexibility training. Pre-heating with hot packs, heat lamps, hot baths or showers, diathermy or massage will increase the effect. These methods may be used before warm-up but not instead of exercises. The heat reduces viscosity and relaxes tissues, which thus offer less resistance to movement. Heat also increases the extensibility of connective and muscle tissue surrounding the joint.

STRENGTH TRAINING

Certain strength training routines can limit joint flexibility. Strength training must be planned to include full-range movements and eccentric work.

In the same way as we overload a muscle in order to increase strength, we must overstretch in order to increase flexibility. The body continually adapts to increasing demand placed upon it, so that moving a joint beyond its existing range and stretching the surrounding tissues will result in increased range as the tissues become more extensible.

USES OF STRETCHING EXERCISES

Stretching exercises should always be included in any exercise scheme. They should be practised after the warm-up in order to enhance performance and reduce the risk of injury. They should be performed during the cool-down to reduce muscle soreness and stiffness. Stretching exercises can also be used as a complete programme, designed progressively to increase the range in all body joints. This type of slow stretch programme allows time for thought and meditation and, as in yoga, pursues a harmony of body, mind and spirit.

METHODS OF STRETCHING

There are various methods of stretching, including ballistic, dynamic, static, proprioceptive neuromuscular facilitation (PNF) and others.

BALLISTIC STRETCHING

This type of stretching involves fast, jerky movements where the increased momentum created by a 'bounce' is used to increase movement at the end of the range, for example bouncing to touch the toes. Ballistics are not generally recommended and should be avoided in class work.

The arguments against their use are physiologically sound:

- A quick or rapid stretch does not allow sufficient time for the tissues to adapt, resulting in strain.
- A sudden jerk applied to a muscle will initiate the stretch reflex and muscle tension will increase. Further pulling against this tension may result in microscopic tears of the myofibrils. Healing will result in the formation of fibrous tissue, which impairs the function of the muscle.

- A quick stretch does not allow for neurological adaptation. Research has shown that the tension generated in a muscle by a fast stretch is far greater than that generated by a slow stretch. Therefore the tensile resistance to fast stretching is much greater.
- Bouncing movements are not easy to control. Therefore the positioning of joints and the direction of movement may not be correct, increasing the likelihood of injury.

Despite all these reasons for not attempting ballistics, some people favour their use for specific training. Gymnasts and dancers may practise them prior to specific actions or routines, but generally they should be avoided.

DYNAMIC STRETCHING

These are movements where a muscle or muscles are worked gradually through their range. Beginning with short-range movements, the actions move progressively through to maximum full range. Dynamic flexibility is required by ball kickers in rugby and soccer, e.g. a gradual stretching of the hamstrings before kicking ensures that the effort of the muscles kicking the ball is not hampered by tight hamstrings. Repetitive free knee extension is performed, increasing the range each time.

STATIC STRETCHING

These are movements which take a muscle slowly and deliberately to the end of its range. The position is then held and further stretch applied. During the holding time, the muscle adapts to the stretch. The stretch reflex controlled by the muscle spindles is inhibited, there is a slow decrease in muscle tension and the muscle relaxes. This allows an increase in muscle length and in the range of joint movement. Research has shown that low-force, long-duration stretching at a raised temperature will result in permanent lengthening.

Static stretching is safer and more effective than ballistic stretching, as the tissues have time to relax. Maximum stretch is achieved when a muscle is fully relaxed and connective tissue is fully stretched. The stretch reflex is inhibited, and so there is no risk of tearing, muscle soreness and damage. Movements are slower, more controlled and more functionally accurate, and there is therefore less risk of injury. Static stretching requires less energy consumption than ballistics.

Static stretching may be classified into active and passive stretching.

- Active stretching is stretching alone, without external aid.

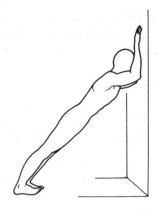

Figure 8.7 *Active stretch for the gastrocnemius*

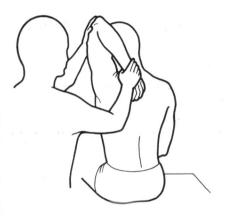

Figure 8.8 *Active assisted stretching of the triceps*

- Active assisted stretching is a stretch performed alone until a limit is reached, at which point a partner helps to gain a further stretch.
- Passive stretching is achieved by an external force such as traction or a partner, while the individual remains inactive.

All static stretching must be controlled and performed with care. Particular care, effective communication and trust must exist between partners in active assisted and passive stretching. These should only be practised by competent, well-trained individuals.

PROPRIOCEPTIVE NEUROMUSCULAR FACILITATION

There are many PNF techniques, which are an excellent way of increasing range of movement, but they require an in-depth knowledge of neurophysiology and are not within the scope of this book. However, one of the techniques, alternate contract/relax, is straightforward and useful, especially following recovery from injury.

This form of increased range is achieved in the following way. A muscle is moved to its point of slight stretch, i.e. at the end of joint movement, and an isometric contraction of that muscle against resistance is performed and held. This is followed by relaxation and further joint movement, which will now be possible.

For example, in prone lying (face down), lift one leg to stretch the hip flexors. Ask a partner to support the leg and to resist an isometric contraction (i.e. not to allow movement as you push down against his or her hand). Relax, then lift the leg higher, as the hip flexors will now allow a greater range of movement.

Alternatively, tilt the head to the left to stretch the right sterno-cleido-mastoid. Now place the hand against the right side of the face. Contract the muscle statically against the hand resistance, hold and relax. The head will now move further to the left.

TECHNIQUES OF STRETCHING

- Select a suitable venue that is warm and well-ventilated. Ensure that there is sufficient space to perform all movements.
- Wear warm clothing to maintain and increase body temperature.
- Check that the floor surface is clean, smooth and non-slip.
- Do not stretch if any of the following contra-indications are present: hyper-mobility, strains or sprains, inflammation of joints, pain in joints, fevers, heart problems, high or low blood pressure, or after a heavy meal.
- Identify the goals (where flexibility is required). Always warm up

with a set of exercises designed to work the large muscle groups. This warm-up will increase muscle temperature, reduce muscle viscosity, decrease muscle tension and promote relaxation and will make tissues more extensible.

- Set the mind into a tranquil and relaxed state.
- Isolate the muscle or group for stretching and place the joint in the correct position. Stretch slowly and evenly, feeling the pull in the belly of the muscle and not at the tendon ends. There should be a feeling of mild discomfort, not pain. Hold the stretch for six to ten seconds to begin with, increasing to 20–30 seconds over time. As the tension decreases, stretch a little further – do not jerk or bounce at the end of the movement. Let pain be the guide. If the pain increases, relax; if the muscle begins to quiver, relax; if muscle tension increases, relax. Move slowly out of the stretch.
- Repeat the stretch five times at the beginning of a programme, eventually working up to ten to fifteen repetitions.
- Exhale as you move into the stretch and relax.
- Stretching programmes should be performed once or twice a day if rapid improvement is required.

THE EFFECTS OF STRETCH TRAINING

The physiological effects of flexibility training are:

- an increased range of movement at joints;
- increased flexibility of the supporting structures;
- increased elasticity and length of muscles;
- reduced tension and increased relaxation in the muscles;
- increased circulation to the muscles;
- improved balance and co-ordination between muscle groups;
- improved posture;
- improved mechanical efficiency and improved speed and skill;
- improved technique and performance, since relaxation of the antagonistic muscles allows the agonist to maximise performance;
- if performed after eccentric work, a reduction of muscle soreness.

DANGERS OF STRETCHING EXERCISES

- Damage to muscles by causing micro-tears of muscle fibres, caused by sudden stretch of cold muscles, or ballistics;
- Damage to joints caused by poor technique;

- Over-stretching of ligaments caused by poor technique or forcing at the end of the range;
- Straining other body areas due to incorrect positioning;
- Raising blood pressure caused by incorrect breathing.

Speed

Speed is the distance moved in a specific time:

$$\text{Speed} = \frac{\text{distance moved}}{\text{time taken}}$$

Speed is a requirement of many activities in athletics and sport. Speed may be required in the lower limbs for sprinting, in the upper limbs for throwing or fast bowling or in both for certain sports such as basketball. Speed is related to muscle strength, flexibility, reaction time and leverage.

STRENGTH

Muscle force is necessary to produce acceleration. The greater the force applied by the muscles, the greater the acceleration and speed. In sprinting, the push-off muscles of the propelling leg will drive the body forward. The greater the strength of these muscles, the greater the driving force. These muscles are the gastrocnemius and soleus in the calf, the quadriceps on the front of the thigh and the gluteus maximus in the buttock. Strengthening exercises for these muscles should form part of the training regime to increase speed. For throwing speed, strengthening exercises are required for the serratus anterior, pectoralis major, anterior deltoid, triceps, wrist and finger extensors.

FLEXIBILITY

A large range of movement at the joints will allow for longer strides, and long fast strides will increase speed. Increased flexibility of the ankle, knee and hip will thus increase running speed. Increased flexibility of the shoulder, elbow and wrist will increase the propulsion force when throwing. Flexibility exercises should therefore be included in training programmes.

REACTION TIME

The ability to react quickly to a stimulus is vital in many sports. Muscles must be able to contract instantly in response to a stimulus such as a starting gun or the hitting of a service ball. Instant reactions to stimuli will improve speed. Reaction time can be improved by repetitive practice of the required action, optimising body position and nervous response. Exercises where a quick response is required, such as ball throwing, catching and running, are also used.

LEVERAGE

Body activities involve the movement of many levers. As previously explained (chapter 6), the levers of the human body are mainly of the third order. These are designed for speed and range of movement. The longer the lever, the greater the speed, providing the force or muscle strength is great enough.

THE EFFECT OF LACTIC ACID ON SPEED

The build-up of lactic acid has an inhibitory effect on muscle contraction. Bursts of fast activity initially use stored ATP and PC, but these are soon used up and fast energy is obtained from the anaerobic breakdown of glycogen into pyruvic acid with the production of lactic acid. This build-up of lactic acid inhibits muscle contraction and therefore reduces speed. Athletes must therefore train to increase their aerobic capacity and to run close to their VO_2max. Since the aerobic metabolism is used for a longer period, there will be little or no lactic acid and little impairment of the muscle action.

This form of anaerobic training will consist initially of short bursts of intense activity for 30–60 seconds and then rests of the same duration. The time is then progressively increased. These activities may include shuttle running or a circuit of set exercises interspersed with running. Training for speed involves different forms of running, beginning with jogging, moving on to running and finishing with maximum-speed sprinting. Variations include maximum-pace running interspersed with walking or jogging. Training must also include specific training at maximum speed for set distances.

Other physical principles affecting speed include reaction forces, friction, resistance forces and mass.

Skill

Skilled movement is balanced, co-ordinated, graceful and precise, with accurate timing and overall rhythmic flow. There is no wastage of energy.

Skill improves as a result of practice and experience. Acquiring a skill is goal-directed: the learner must be aware of the desired end result and how to achieve it. Constant repetitions of patterns of movement must be practised until they are registered in the brain and can eventually be performed automatically (see chapter 14). In order to master an activity and give a skilled performance, the activity should be broken down into small chunks or parts. Each part should be practised until a satisfactory standard is achieved. The sequence of movements is then linked, and the complete activity is practised until all errors are eliminated and the performance is automatic. Muscle strength and flexibility contribute to a skilled performance, but other factors are involved, such as neuro-muscular co-ordination, balance, etc.

Balance will improve by gradually reducing stability. Practice of a movement should begin in a stable position and progress to a less stable position. The speed of performance can also vary from normal to slow and then fast. Rhythm and timing will improve as the activity is mastered and co-ordination, grace and precision are achieved.

Nutrition and diet

This is a vast and specialised field, which is not within the scope of this book. However, there are basic facts that are worth noting.

Everyone requires a good, balanced diet for maintaining health and fitness. Nutrients are chemicals used by the body to provide energy, to build new tissues and to carry out various functions or processes. Athletes and sports people must carefully consider their diet in order to meet the demands for the extra energy required in training and competition.

Six basic nutrients are necessary for a healthy diet. These are carbohydrates, fats (lipids), proteins, vitamins, minerals and water. Fibre is an additional requirement, as it aids the functioning of the digestive tract.

CARBOHYDRATES

These give the body its primary source of energy. Carbohydrates are the starches, sugars and cellulose found in pulses, cereals, bread, potatoes, pasta and root vegetables. During digestion complex sugars (polysaccharides) are broken down into disaccharides and then to monosaccharides, i.e. glucose and fructose. If the glucose is not required immediately for energy it is converted by the liver to glycogen. Glycogen is then stored in the liver or in the muscle tissue cells. If these stores are full, the liver will change the glucose into fat, which is stored in adipose tissue. Fast, short-duration sprints use carbohydrate only as the fuel for muscle contraction. Medium-pace, moderate activities, such as jogging, use carbohydrates first and then move into using fats.

FATS

Fats are the body's secondary source of energy. Fats or lipids are obtained from animal and vegetable sources. They are found in butter, milk, cheese, meat and so on, and in soya beans, nuts, olives, avocados, etc. During digestion, fats are broken down into fatty acids and glycerol. If they are not required for immediate energy, they are stored in adipose tissue and in the liver. Some lipids are used to resynthesise tissues such as the myelin sheath of certain nerves and thromboplastin for blood clotting. A high fat intake increases the likelihood of developing high cholesterol levels, hypertension and heart disease. Although fats produce twice the amount of energy as that obtained from carbohydrates, they are the body's secondary source because they are more difficult to break down to meet a demand for energy: carbohydrates will be used first and then fat. Endurance activities use fats as an energy source. As well as providing energy, fat acts as an insulator, conserving body heat.

PROTEINS

Proteins are used for tissue repair, growth and body-building. Proteins are obtained from food products such as meat, fish, eggs, milk, cheese, peas, beans and pulses. During digestion they are broken down into amino acids. They are used for the repair and growth of keratin, collagen and elastin. They are also used for the production of actin and myosin and therefore for the increase in size of myofibrils. Proteins are needed to repair damage following bone fractures, muscle strain or tears of ligaments. They are used for making antibodies, enzymes and hormones. Proteins are only used as an energy source in cases of starvation or very long-distance running when all stores of carbohydrates and fats have been used up.

VITAMINS

Vitamins are required to maintain growth and metabolism. A large range of vitamins is obtained from food sources, and a balanced diet is essential to ensure adequate intake. Few vitamins can be synthesised in the body, but exceptions are the vitamins K and B6. Some are stored in the body, but others are eliminated in the urine.

A deficiency of vitamins can result in various disorders and diseases, such as rickets, beriberi, neuritis, pernicious anaemia and scurvy.

MINERALS

A number of elements are essential for regulating and maintaining life processes. Calcium is required for the formation of bones and teeth, blood clotting and the conduction of nerve impulses. Iron is required as a component of haemoglobin and muscle myoglobin.

WATER

Water is essential for the functioning of body processes. It has many functions: it lubricates, it dissolves substances and it is found bathing all tissue cells. It facilitates the transportation of nutrients and oxygen from the blood into the cells and the transfer of waste products from cells to the blood. As blood plasma (90 per cent of which is water), it transports substances around the body. It cools the body by evaporation and so helps to regulate body temperature. Two to three litres of water or fruit juice should be drunk every day. This is in addition to any tea, coffee or alcohol consumed as these are diuretics, which increase fluid loss.

Under normal conditions the body maintains a balance between fluid intake and output. However, during and following exercise a great deal of body heat is generated by the contraction of muscles. This must be reduced through evaporation (sweating), which causes a loss of water. This water must be replaced during and after prolonged exercise, particularly in hot weather, as dehydration may occur. Concentrated, dark urine is an indication of dehydration, while pale, dilute urine indicates a sufficient intake of water. With dehydration blood volume is reduced, and this can affect the performance of exercise as there is less blood available for the heart to pump to the muscles. This affects their ability to contract to maximum effect, and muscle cramps and 'stitches' may result. Drinking water alone may not be enough to rehydrate the body, as this interferes with electrolytic balance and urine output is increased before rehydration is complete. Sports drinks have now been developed that contain sodium and/or carbohydrate. The desirability and effectiveness of these drinks is still controversial and research continues. Many nutritionists believe that the diet of most people is already too high in sodium and, therefore, that it is not necessary to provide added intake in drinks. It must also be remembered that carbohydrates supply calories, so anyone wishing to control weight will not require the extra calories found in these drinks.

FIBRE

Fibre provides roughage and bulk, which stimulates peristalsis and facilitates the movement of waste through the digestive tract. Thus, waste passes more quickly and efficiently through the large intestine for excretion. A high-fibre diet must be accompanied by a high fluid intake in order to keep the colon functioning efficiently.

WEIGHT CONTROL

The food we eat provides the energy for bodily functions. The *metabolic rate* is the rate at which the body uses fuel. Weight control is largely a balance between energy input (food eaten) and energy output (energy used).

- If energy input equals energy output weight remains stable (weight is neither gained nor lost).
- If energy input is greater than energy output, weight increases as the excess fuel is stored in the body as fat.
- If energy input is less than energy output, weight is lost as fuel is taken from the fat stores.

Therefore the most effective way to lose weight is to eat less and increase the level of activity.

Aerobic exercise is the most effective form of activity for losing weight, as it utilises fat as well as carbohydrate for energy.

Research has shown that fancy 'miracle' or 'magic' diets do not work and are harmful to health. The body reacts to starvation by reducing the metabolic rate in order to ensure survival. Therefore, during rapid weight-loss diets energy output is considerably reduced. When normal eating is resumed weight is gained quickly. This results in weight loss followed by weight gain – the 'yo-yo effect'.

Any diet should aim at reducing weight by around 1 kg per week. It is important to eat healthily and to include each of the foods necessary for health, but it is worth noting that:

1 gram of carbohydrate provides	17 kilojoules (4 calories) of energy
1 gram of protein provides	17 kilojoules (4 calories) of energy
but	
1 gram of fat provides	39 kilojoules (9 calories) of energy.

Therefore, eating more carbohydrate and protein and cutting down on fat will result in a lower energy intake and a more rapid weight loss.

Body composition

This divides the body into two components: fat and fat-free mass (FFM). The ratio of fat to muscle tissue is also an important factor in weight control. The percentage of body fat can be influenced by heredity, body type and the number of fat cells that developed in the first two years of life. On average, females have about 30–50 per cent more fat than males.

- *Endomorphs* are short, curvaceous and plump.
- *Ectomorphs* are long-limbed and slim.
- *Mesomorphs* are muscular and stocky.

Muscle tissue has a high metabolic rate, so it is an advantage to have a high proportion of muscle tissue in the body. The metabolic rate will be higher and fuel will be used more efficiently. It is a disadvantage to have a high percentage of fat on the body, a condition known as obesity.

A high percentage of body fat increases the risk of developing many serious health problems. These include:

- cardio-vascular disease and strokes
- hypertension
- varicose veins
- diabetes mellitus
- kidney disease
- gall bladder problems
- cirrhosis of the liver
- high cholesterol levels

- back problems and joint problems due to increased stress
- osteoarthritis

Exercise of all varieties will increase the metabolic rate, but research indicates that aerobic activities are the most effective for losing fat. The desirable level of fat for men is 12–20 per cent. The desirable level of fat for women is 20–30 per cent. Male athletes may carry as little as 5 per cent and female athletes 16 per cent.

A GUIDE TO HEALTHY EATING

- Reduce the intake of fat, particularly animal fat.
- Reduce the intake of red meat, as it has a high fat content.
- Reduce the intake of sugar and salt.
- Eat plenty of fish, particularly oily fish such as mackerel, salmon, herring and trout.
- Eat plenty of fresh or frozen vegetables (do not overcook).
- Eat plenty of fresh, frozen or dried fruit.
- Eat wholemeal foods such as bread, pasta, rice, cereals, pulses and beans.
- Eat a wide variety of foods.
- Cut down on alcohol.
- Eat plenty of fibre.
- Drink two to three litres of water per day.
- A low-fat, high-carbohydrate and moderate-protein diet is recommended.

CHAPTER 9

Relaxation and posture

Relaxation

Relaxation means freedom from tension and anxiety and involves both a physiological and a psychological state. Tension and anxiety are caused by stress, which upsets the body balance, known as homeostasis. The body ceases to function efficiently, resulting in lethargy, illness and disease.

Stress has been defined as a non-specific response of the body to any demand made on it. Stressors, those factors causing stress, may be extrinsic or intrinsic. They may be social, chemical, bacterial, physical, climatic or psychological. People differ in their ability to cope with stress; some are more affected than others. The symptoms of stress are easily identifiable: increased sweating, increased heart rate, higher blood pressure, rapid breathing, dryness of the mouth, inability to cope, feeling overwhelmed and out of control, inability to concentrate or make decisions, trembling, nail biting, frequent urination, non-stop talking, pacing and other nervous habits.

It is impossible to remove all stressors from daily life. Indeed, a certain degree of stress is desirable and productive, and it can produce feelings of thrill and excitement. The ability to relax combats stress and reduces its harmful effects. It conserves energy, reduces fatigue, lethargy and overtiredness and helps the body to return to a state of homeostasis.

Allowing the body to rest and recover is essential for those participating in gymnastics, athletics, sport and fitness activities. It is important for all participants in these activities to practise and master relaxation techniques, since the ability to relax at the right moment can improve performance. Total relaxation conserves energy and concentrates the mind before events and so should be practised both before events and during breaks or intervals.

AIDS TO RELAXATION

A variety of aids can be used to promote relaxation:

- heat therapy, e.g. heat packs, heat blankets, hot baths, showers, sauna and steam baths and infra-red lamps;
- cold therapy, e.g. cold packs and wraps;
- massage performed in a deep, slow and rhythmic manner;
- preparations such as analgesic liniments, wintergreen and other muscle relaxants.

RELAXATION TECHNIQUES

To achieve long-term benefits, the individual must learn to recognise the difference between being in a tense state and being in a relaxed state. As physical and mental relaxation are interdependent, both must be taught. Although relaxation techniques may appear simple, they are skills that must be learned and practised regularly.

Examples of relaxation techniques:

- The relaxation response
- Progressive relaxation (contract/relax technique)
- Visualisation or imagery
- Biofeedback.

Regardless of the technique, the selection of a warm, quiet environment and the positioning and comfort of the client are important considerations. These factors alone may be sufficient to elicit the relaxation response, as explained below.

PREPARATION OF THE ROOM

- The area should be warm and well ventilated.
- The area should be quiet and away from any distracting noises or activities.
- The lighting should be low and diffused.
- The colour scheme should be soft and warming, using pastel colours rather than harsh, bold colours.
- The area should be spotlessly clean and tidy. All linen and towels should be boil-washed and well laundered.
- A comfortable mattress on the floor provides the best support, with pillows for the head and knees. Two low plinths pushed together and covered with a thin mattress can be used. (Clients feel more secure nearer the ground and on a wide rather than a narrow surface.)

- Light blankets can be used for additional warmth.
- Very soft relaxing music may be played in the background. This depends on client preference, as some clients do not like absolute quiet and become tense.

CLIENT CARE

A full client consultation should be carried out.

- Allow the client time to discuss their lifestyle and any problems that may be contributing to stress and anxiety levels.
- Discuss stress levels at work or during sport or training that may be affecting performance. Advise and suggest strategies for coping where possible. Explain how relaxation will help.
- Suggest suitable clothing, such as a loose-fitting cotton vest, T-shirt or sweater and loose-fitting pyjama or track suit bottoms. Loose socks can be worn on the feet. (Do not allow the client to walk around in socks as there is a danger of slipping.)
- If suitable clothing is not available, loosen the clothing, remove the tie and belt, loosen the collar and trousers or skirt and remove the shoes.
- Suggest that the client uses the toilet, as it is impossible to relax with a full bladder.
- Use some form of heat, if available, prior to the commencement of relaxation training. (Follow the correct procedure when applying heat.)
- Create an atmosphere conducive to relaxation. Smile, be calm, pleasant and relaxed, speak slowly and clearly, keep your voice low and do not rush or hurry the client. Explain the procedure clearly and carefully to alleviate any anxiety.

THE RELAXATION RESPONSE

The client relaxes in response to four basic conditions:

- a quiet environment – this cuts out noise, limits distraction and allows the individual to switch off;
- a comfortable position – the position selected for all relaxation techniques is very important. The position should be selected to suit the preference of the client: lying, half lying or the recovery position may be chosen. The body must be well supported with pillows to minimise muscle effort and to enable the client to remain in this position for a considerable length of time;
- mental concentration – this can be an image on which to concentrate, such as a sphere, box or vase, or any object in the room, such as a clock or mirror. The client concentrates hard

on this one image and empties the mind of other thoughts or images;

- a passive attitude – this is the most difficult, especially for those with extreme mental anxiety. It involves letting go and emptying the mind of thoughts and distractions.

PROGRESSIVE RELAXATION

This method was developed by Dr. Edmund Jacobson, one of the pioneers in the field of relaxation. It aims to develop an awareness of the difference between feelings of tension and relaxation within muscles and muscle groups. The client is taught to contract and relax each muscle group in sequence, from the foot to the head. With practice, the client will appreciate the difference between being tense and relaxed and will develop the ability to adopt the relaxed state quickly. The client can then be taught to recognise differing degrees of tension within muscles by using the same sequence but varying the contraction, from full contraction to part contraction and minimal contraction, for each muscle or group.

The therapist should select a suitable venue and prepare the client (see page 123). The client should lie on a mattress and be fully supported. Modifications of the lying position can be used, for example the recovery position, with the body well supported with pillows, the supine position (on the back) with a pillow under the head and knees, or half lying, with pillows for the head and knees. Encourage the client to 'let go', breathe deeply and close the eyes gently.

The technique is then practised as follows, beginning with the feet and repeating each movement three times:

- Pull the feet up hard (dorsi-flexion), then let go.
- Push the feet down hard (plantar flexion), then let go.
- Push the knees down hard against the floor, then let go.
- Push the leg down hard against the floor, then let go.
- Tighten the buttock muscles hard, then let go.
- Pull the abdominal muscles in hard, then let go.
- Raise the shoulders off the floor, then let go.
- Press the shoulders hard into the floor, then let go.
- Press the arms hard into the floor, then let go.
- Curl the fingers to make a fist, then let go.
- Press the head into the floor, then let go.
- Screw up and tighten the face, then let go.
- Tighten all groups, then let go.

The client should breathe out as he or she 'lets go'.

The therapist must use her voice to good effect when teaching relaxation. The command 'tighten hard' should be firm, and 'let go' should be spoken in a lower tone and drawn out longer to encourage the feeling of letting go. The terms 'relax' and 'release' can be used or interchanged with 'let go'.

Clients can then practise the sequence on their own until they are free of tension and sleepy. They should be left for fifteen to twenty minutes and then woken up slowly.

As clients develop the ability they can be taught to appreciate differing degrees of tension. This is done in the same way as above, except that the first contraction should be maximal, the second contraction partial and the third contraction minimal. The commands would be as follows:

- Pull the feet up hard, and relax.
- Gently pull the feet up, just feel the muscle pulling, and relax.
- Move the foot upwards ever so slightly, and relax.

Clients should then practise the three different contractions in their own time, feeling the difference in muscle tension each time.

The therapist will work through the body in this way, using the same sequence as above.

TASKS

Work with a partner.

- Position your partner comfortably in the recovery position, using pillows as required.

- Teach your partner to relax using the progressive relaxation technique.

VISUALISATION OR IMAGERY

This technique requires the individual to visualise situations or conditions conducive to relaxation. For example:

- Imagine lying on the beach in warm sunshine. It is quiet and peaceful, you feel warm and heavy.
- Imagine lying in a field in warm sunshine. You smell the grass. You feel warm and heavy.
- Imagine sinking into a feather duvet. It feels soft and warm and wraps around you.
- Think of any situation that recalls warmth, comfort and peace.
- Concentrate entirely on the rhythm of breathing, letting the breathing become deeper and slower.

Any examples that enhance relaxation can be included.

Visualisation with breathing can be used to good effect when performing static-stretch and flexibility exercises that require the relaxed state.

The client should exhale and move into the stretch position, stretching until tension is felt in the muscle belly. This position is held while the client breathes in and out slowly for a few cycles. The client then breathes in then out slowly while moving into a further stretch, imagining the muscle fibres letting go and lengthening. When tension develops the position is held briefly, followed by relaxation.

BIOFEEDBACK

When it is difficult to appreciate the difference between muscle tension and relaxation, biofeedback techniques using special equipment may be applied. The equipment gives a reading that relates to the degree of tension, and the mind is then used to attempt a change in the reading.

Posture

Posture is the term used to describe the alignment of the body, in other words how the body is held. Good posture means that the body is balanced and the muscle work required to maintain an upright position is minimal. Poor posture means that the body is out of balance and certain muscles must contract strongly to maintain this position. Over time, this means that those muscles will tighten and shorten, while others weaken and stretch. This muscle imbalance imposes stresses on the underlying structures, the ligaments and joints, resulting in deformities, stiffness and pain. The body loses its ability to function at maximum efficiency and the performance of everyday activities, movement and exercise can become severely limited.

Poor alignment of one part of the body can affect other parts. This can be more clearly understood if we think of the body in terms of segments. Each segment must be perfectly balanced on the one below. If one segment moves forwards, backwards or sideways, adjustments have to be made in all the other segments for balance to be restored.

Posture is dynamic, constantly adjusting to counteract the forces acting upon the body. Postural adjustments may be made consciously or unconsciously. The cerebral cortex, basal nuclei, cerebellum and brain stem all play a part in the control of posture.

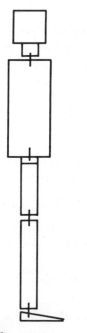

Figure 9.1 *Body segments must be balanced one on the other*

These higher centres respond to different impulses arriving from various sensory receptors. Information on the body's position in space is received from muscle spindles, from tendon and joint receptors, from the eyes and ears and from the skin on the soles of the feet. The higher centres respond to incoming information and relay impulses back to the muscles, initiating muscle contraction to produce corrective action.

Posture is influenced by many factors, both physical and psychological. A large proportion of the population leads a sedentary life and takes little exercise, which leads to muscle imbalance and poor body alignment. Other factors that influence posture include heredity, weight distribution, height, nervous tension, illness, fatigue, occupational stress, poor working conditions and poor sitting positions. Psychological and emotional states also have an effect – people who are happy, confident and extrovert, with high self-esteem, exhibit good posture, while those who are unhappy, sad, introverted and lacking in confidence, with low self-esteem, have poor posture.

Poor posture results in muscle imbalance. Some muscles become tight, while others will be overstretched. This imposes stress on the ligaments, tendons and underlying joints, producing pain and stiffness. In addition, certain muscles are unable to work through their full range. This not only restricts the activities of daily living but severely limits the capacity to perform at maximum potential in athletics, sports, dancing, etc.

Poor posture affects general health. The natural movements of the thorax may be restricted and its expansion limited, which results in shallow breathing. This reduces the intake of oxygen and the elimination of carbon dioxide. The circulation is affected due to the tension in muscles and the reduction in thoracic movement, which mean that blood is unable to flow freely around the body. This limits the delivery of nutrients and the elimination of waste products.

Good postural habits should be developed when young and maintained throughout life. It is possible to improve posture for all age groups through appropriate exercise. The extent of the improvement will depend on the degree of deformity, the age and the commitment of the individual.

Good posture is important for the following reasons:

- maintaining muscle balance;
- improving body shape and appearance;
- preventing muscle tension, spasm and pain;
- preventing stresses on ligaments, tendons and joints;

- preventing skeletal deformities and associated pain;
- increasing the movement of the thorax, resulting in deeper breathing with an increase in oxygen intake and the elimination of carbon dioxide;
- improving the efficiency of the circulatory system;
- improving the performance of all activities and exercises and enhancing peak performance;
- reducing the risk of musculo-skeletal injuries.

Evaluation of posture

Posture must be accurately examined and evaluated before correction can take place. An accurate assessment of posture should form part of the client consultation. All findings should be carefully recorded and appropriate exercises devised for correction of the faults.

AIDS TO POSTURAL ASSESSMENT

The following aids can be used to make assessment easier and more accurate.

- a plumb line to check body alignment (see chapter 6);
- a mirror to provide visual feedback for the client. First, look at the client's normal posture and discuss any problem areas. Correct the posture and discuss the improvements. View the posture from the front, side and back. On the front view, lines can be drawn to check the level of the ear lobes and shoulders, the waist angles, and the level of the right and left anterior superior iliac spines and the knees. On the side view, draw a vertical line from the ear lobe to just in front of the lateral malleolus – does it fall through the plumb-line points? Check for round shoulders, kyphosis, lordosis, flat back, sway back and hyper-extended knees. On the back view, check for winged scapulae, scoliosis, pelvic level and buttock folds.
- a graphed board – the client stands in front of the board and the relevant bony points (ear lobes, shoulders, waist angles, knees) are marked, examined for any deviation and discussed.

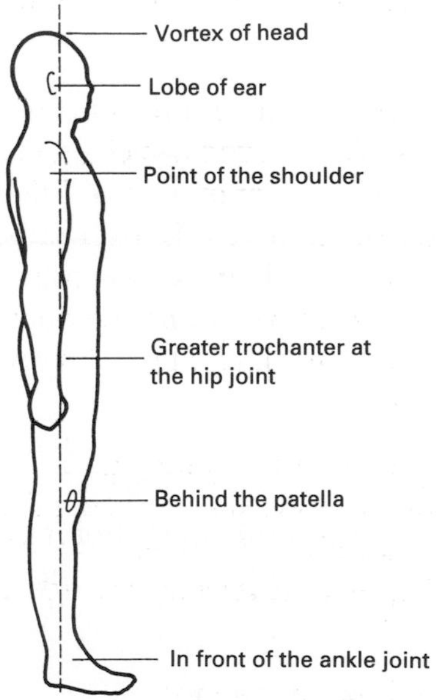
Vortex of head
Lobe of ear
Point of the shoulder
Greater trochanter at the hip joint
Behind the patella
In front of the ankle joint
Figure 9.2 *Points that the line of gravity will pass through when posture is correct*

It is not necessary to use all these aids, but one or two will help the client to appreciate his or her problems.

PROCEDURE

- Welcome and observe the client as she/he walks into the room.
- Ask the client to sit, observing how he or she sits down.
- Take the client's details – name, address, doctor's address,

medical history, occupation. Discuss fully any stresses at work, working positions, seating, etc. Discuss lifestyle, associated activities, and nutritional standards. Try to assess the client's psychological state while talking – is he or she tense, under stress, fatigued or exhausted? Is the client an introvert or extrovert, or are there any other factors that might influence posture?

● Ask the client to undress down to pants only, making sure that there is complete privacy.

● If possible observe the posture as the client walks around the room (this may not be possible in a small cubicle). Many problems can be observed when the body is in motion. Observe the client sitting down and standing up: are the movements evenly balanced or does he or she sit and stand unevenly?

● Ask the client to adopt a normal stance and assess the posture from the front, side and back.

● Discuss any problem areas with the client. Stand him or her in front of a mirror, indicate the postural faults and show how they may be corrected.

● Correct the client's posture and ask him or her to hold the adjustments until good posture is obtained (the new positioning will seem very unnatural at first).

● Tell the client to relax and then to make the adjustments independently and hold the corrected stance.

● Explain to the client that frequent practice is needed throughout the day.

● Teach appropriate exercises to restore muscle balance.

THE EXAMINATION OF POSTURE

FROM THE FRONT

Head position:

● Are the ear lobes level? If they are not there is muscle imbalance. The sterno-cleido-mastoid and the upper fibres of the trapezius are tight on the lower side, while those on the other side will be stretched.

Shoulders:

● Are they level, or is one higher than the other, indicating muscle imbalance? The upper fibres of the trapezius and levator scapulae are tight on the raised side. A difference in level may also indicate scoliosis, so check for that also. (A slight difference is considered normal.)

- Are both shoulders held high? This indicates tension in the muscles on both sides. The right and left upper fibres of the trapezius and the levator scapulae are tight.
- Are the shoulders drawn forwards, rounded? This indicates muscle imbalance. The pectoral muscles are tight but the middle fibres of the trapezius and the rhomboids are stretched.
- Are there hollows above the clavicles? This indicates muscle tension, which may be due to respiratory problems such as asthma.

Breasts:

- Are the breasts held high or sagging? If there is breast sag and round shoulders, correction of the posture may help to lift the breasts.

Waist:

- Are the waist angles on the right and left level? If one is lower than the other, there may be spinal deformity or a difference in leg length.

Anterior superior iliac spines:

- Are they level? If not, there may be spinal deformity or a difference in leg length.
- Are they dropped forward? This indicates a lordosis with a tight erector spinae and quadratus lumborum and weak abdominals.
- Are they dropped backwards? This indicates a flat back or sway back, with weak back extensors, i.e. the erector spinae and quadratus lumborum, and tight abdominals.

Patellae:

- Do they point forwards? If not there may be knock knees (genu valgum) or bow legs (genu varum).

Toes:

- Do they point forwards? If they point outwards there may be flattening of the medial arch and flat feet.
- If they point inwards or outwards, the weight distribution over the foot will be wrong, causing foot problems.
- Look for bunions, where the big toe deviates towards and sometimes across the other toes and there is swelling at the metatarso-phalangeal joint.
- Look for hammer toes, where the inter-phalangeal joints are deformed.

FROM THE SIDE

Use a plumb line. This should fall through the lobe of the ear, the point of the shoulder and the hip joint, behind the patella and just in front of the lateral malleolus.

Head position:

- Is the neck or cervical curve exaggerated and the chin forward? This means that the neck extensors, the upper fibres of the trapezius at the back of the neck, are tight and the neck flexors are weak.

Thoracic curve:

- Is there kyphosis, i.e. an exaggerated thoracic curve, giving a humped look? This means that the pectoral muscles are tight and the middle fibres of the trapezius and rhomboids are weak.

Abdomen:

- Is the abdomen protruding or sagging forwards, indicating weakness of the abdominal muscles? The pelvis may be tilted forward.

Lumbar curve:

- Is there lordosis, i.e. an exaggerated lumbar curve with the spine curved inwards? This means that there will be an anterior pelvic tilt with weak abdominals and a tight erector spinae and quadratus lumborum.
- If the lumbar region is flat, which is much less common, the erector spinae and quadratus lumborum will be weak.

Buttocks:

- Are the buttocks well toned with strong muscles, or are the gluteal muscles weak and sagging?

Knees:

- Are the knees hyper-extended?

FROM THE BACK

Head:

- Are the ear lobes level or is the head tilted, indicating muscle imbalance? (See front.)

Shoulders:

- Are they level? (See front.)
- Are there winged scapulae, i.e. the inferior angle and medial border of the scapulae lift away from the chest wall? This

indicates a weakness of the serratus anterior and the lower fibres of the trapezius.

Spine:

- Is there scoliosis, i.e. a lateral deviation of the spine? This may be an S or C curve to the right or left. If you are unsure, pull a finger firmly down the spinous processes: the red line should be straight, and will show up any deviation. A scoliosis may be structural (present from birth). Or it may be postural, and will straighten out when the body is flexed forward.

Buttocks:

- Are the buttock folds level? If they are not, scoliosis, lateral pelvic tilt or different leg length may be present.

Heels:

- Are these square and firmly planted on the ground? If not, the weight distribution will be uneven.

CORRECTION OF THE POSTURE

The correction of the posture should begin at the feet. Each position should be maintained as the subsequent one is practised.

FEET

Stand with the feet four to six inches apart, with the toes pointing forward. The weight should be evenly distributed between the balls of the feet and the heels.

Practise the following:

- Raise the toes off the ground, feel the weight evenly distributed between the balls and heels, then lower the toes.
- Sway the body forwards, feeling more weight on the balls.
- Sway the body backwards, feeling more weight on the heels.
- Position the body so that the weight is evenly distributed between the balls and the heels. Lift the medial arch slightly, but do not curl the toes.

KNEES

- Press the knees backwards hard, ease the knees by bending them slightly, then find the mid-point and pull the kneecaps upwards by tightening the quadriceps muscle.
- If the knees are hyper-extended, ease them slightly and pull the kneecaps upwards as above.

- If the knees are bowed or knock-kneed, tighten the kneecaps, rotate the thighs outwards and tighten the buttocks to bring the kneecaps to point forward.

Check the feet again after performing these movements.

PELVIS

Tilt the pelvis forwards and then backwards; pull it forwards again slightly, tucking the tail under, and hold this balance. Pull the abdomen in and breathe out as the pelvis is pulled forward, then hold this position while breathing normally.

THORAX

Pull the thorax upwards from the waist as you breathe in, drawing the shoulders backwards and downwards. Hold this position while breathing normally. Do not thrust the chest forwards.

NECK AND HEAD

Elongate the neck and pull the chin backwards. Feel as though someone is pulling the hair upwards at the crown.

Check the feet, knees, pelvis and thorax again, hold this position and then relax.

Practise this correction several times a day and during various activities; correct the posture during inhalation and hold the balance during exhalation.

If the new posture is maintained while walking around, it will eventually become habitual.

T A S K S

Work with a partner. Carry out a role play with one of you as the client and one as the therapist.

- Greet the client and carry out a consultation.

- Assess the posture using the plumb line.
- Teach the correction of the posture.

PART C Assessment and exercise

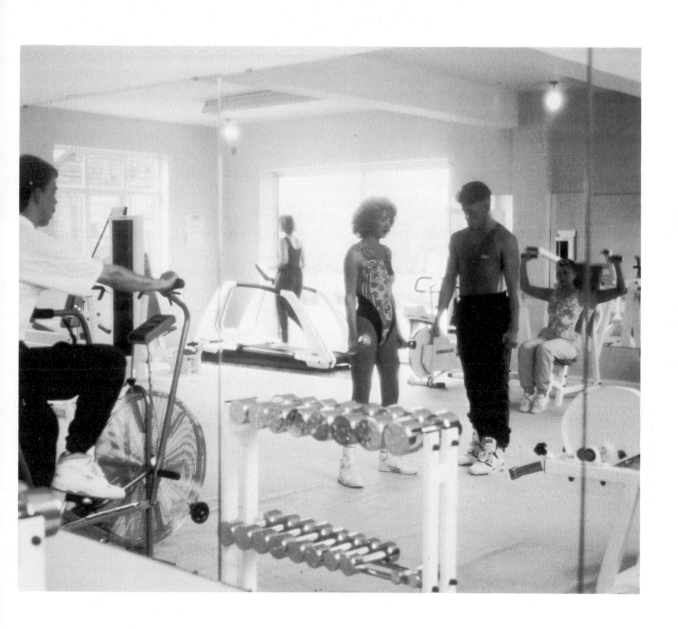

Introduction – important points to remember

- To improve fitness, the principle of overload must be applied. Exercises must become progressively harder. Repeating the same exercise a set number of times will maintain a level of fitness but will not result in significant improvement. The variables that are used to increase overload are *intensity*, *duration* and *frequency*.

- Different types of exercise stress different body systems and produce different effects. Cardio-respiratory or aerobic endurance is a fundamental requirement of fitness for everyone. Other components should be specific to the sport or performance and meet the needs of the individual.

- Muscle flexibility and the range of joint movement will improve through regular stretching exercises.

- Muscle strength and bulk will increase through strengthening exercises, i.e. regularly working the muscle against resistance. The degree of tension developed in a muscle will be directly proportional to the overload. Fewer repetitions at maximum overload will increase muscle strength.

- Muscle endurance, i.e. the capacity of a muscle to repeat an activity without fatigue, will improve if the muscle is made to perform repetitive movements. High repetitions with low resistance will increase muscle endurance.

- Speed will increase if movements and activities are practised at increasing pace.

- Skill, agility, balance and co-ordination develop through repeated practice of an activity, increasing the difficulty by altering the base, the centre of gravity and the pace.

- Cardio-respiratory endurance will improve in response to regular practice of aerobic activities such as jogging, walking, cycling, swimming and aerobic exercise classes. The exercises must be slow and steady and increase very gradually in intensity. This allows the heart, blood vessels and lungs to deliver sufficient oxygen to the muscles for the oxidation of glucose. If the exercises become too fast or intense, then anaerobic metabolism takes over.

- To develop aerobic endurance, the heart rate must be raised, but it must not be raised beyond 80–85 per cent of an individual's maximum heart rate. Remember: MHR is calculated as 220 minus the person's age. Initially, the pulse rate should be raised to only 60 per cent of MHR, progressing to 70 per cent and then to 80–85 per cent. The elevated heart rate must be maintained for fifteen to twenty minutes per session. Exercise should be repeated three to four times per week on alternate days to allow time for recovery.

- To develop anaerobic systems, short sharp bursts of activity must be practised. These should be explosive and dynamic activities such as squash, fast sprints, shot putting, etc.

- Spot reduction of fat through exercise is *not* possible. Exercising a specific area of the body will improve muscle tone in that area, but will not disperse covering fat. To reduce body fat, calories consumed (intake) must be less than calories used (output). Only then is fat removed from all over the body and broken down for energy. Aerobic exercises are high calorie burners, use fat for energy and are the best way of reducing body fat. Strengthening exercises are low calorie burners, so lots of curl-ups will not remove fat from the abdomen, although they will improve the strength of abdominal muscles.

- Weight is often gained rather than lost when people take up exercise, even though fat is reduced. This is because muscle tissue is heavier than fat. Losing weight is not an indication of fitness: it is the ratio of fat to muscle that is important. More muscle and less fat will result in an increase in fitness and better body shape.

- Muscle tissue has a high metabolic rate. Therefore having more muscle tissue gives an individual a higher basic metabolic rate, which means that calories are burnt up more quickly. This makes it easier to lose weight. Through regular exercise people who burn calories slowly can become high calorie burners, thus reducing fat stores more rapidly.

- Muscles will not change to fat if exercising stops, as is commonly supposed. However, muscle strength will be reduced and the muscles will feel softer. Muscle and fat are completely different tissues. Fat is stored on the body as a reserve of energy if calorific intake is greater than calorific output.

- The warm-up is a very important part of all training and exercise routines. It enables the energy systems to increase their rate of work gradually. It warms muscles, which improves their contractability and flexibility. It improves the flexibility of connective tissue components and reduces the likelihood of injury. The warm-up should include mobilising exercises, pulse-raising exercises and simple stretch.

- The cool-down or warm-down is equally important, as it allows the system to slow down gradually and aids the removal of the waste products lactic acid and carbon dioxide. The cool-down enables the body to return to a stable state, i.e. homeostasis is re-established.

- Exercises should never stop suddenly, nor should one stand still after vigorous exercise, as fainting and dizziness may result. During vigorous exercise the blood vessels supplying the muscles dilate, which increases the load on the heart, but the contracting muscles assist in pumping the blood around the body. If exercise stops suddenly, the vessels are still dilated and blood pools in the legs due to gravitational pull. This deprives the brain of oxygen, causing dizziness and faintness. The pressure on the heart is increased as it attempts to maintain blood supply. The cool-down must include gentle jogging or walking around, or stretching and breathing exercises that are performed while lying down.

CHAPTER 10

Safety and hygiene factors related to exercise

Contra-indications to exercise

All clients should have a thorough consultation before embarking on an exercise programme. Any of the following conditions would indicate that the client should not exercise. Unfamiliar conditions may be highlighted during consultation. If in doubt, always seek medical advice.

Common contra-indications are:

- any recent injuries: these would include fractures, strains, sprains, ruptures or tears. It is sometimes desirable to maintain fitness in other parts of the body while the injured part is immobilised. The exercises for other body parts must be carefully planned and performed, ensuring that no stress is placed on the injured part and surrounding tissues;

- heart conditions or any history of heart disease. Appropriate exercise regimes are undertaken following heart attacks and surgery, but these should be medically directed or supervised;

- high blood pressure: generally, if the blood pressure is controlled by drugs, exercise is allowed, but check with the client's doctor. Relaxation can help hypertensive clients, but isometrics should never be performed;

- any acute fevers, such as influenza, glandular fever, the common cold, etc;

- any infections, such as throat infections, measles, chicken pox, etc;

- any inflammatory joint conditions, such as arthritis. Rheumatoid arthritis is a systemic condition in which joints become hot, swollen and stiff. Osteoarthritis is a condition of wear of the joints and the cartilage wears thin, making movement very painful;

- any neurological disorders, such as strokes, multiple sclerosis, etc. – exercises for these conditions must be medically supervised;
- any other undiagnosed illness: seek a doctor's advice;
- any musculo-skeletal problems, such as joint or back pain;
- pain and soreness in muscles caused by trauma or injury as opposed to delayed onset of muscle stiffness;
- during pregnancy medical consent must be sought and gentle exercises only should be given. During the first three months of pregnancy, particular care must be taken. The fit client who has exercised regularly may continue with low-impact, low-intensity work. Weights should not be used, nor should exercises that increase intra-abdominal pressure be performed.
- after eating a heavy meal or under the influence of alcohol;
- if overtired or exhausted;
- if under the influence of pain-killing drugs;
- if there has been any past difficulty with exercise.

Be particularly aware of increasing problems with age. To be safe, all those over 40 should have a medical check-up before starting an exercise programme. Those who are at greatest risk are:

- obese people;
- those with a history of heart problems in the immediate family;
- hypertensives;
- diabetics – a doctor's referral is important, especially if the client is on insulin;
- those with a history of lung problems, such as asthma, bronchitis or emphysema;
- smokers.

Refer these people for a check-up before commencing exercise programmes.

Safety factors to observe while exercising

THE PREMISES

- The room should be warm, well ventilated and without draughts.
- There must be good, even lighting, with no pools of light or dark corners.

- Lights should be shielded with guards, particularly if games are played.
- The floor should be firm, smooth and non-slip, and preferably sprung.
- There must be sufficient space for everyone to move freely, with no overcrowding.
- The room should be clean and uncluttered; all apparatus not in use should be stored neatly away from the working area.
- Apparatus should be in good condition; there should be no rough edges or sharp protruding parts that could cause injury.
- There must be a sufficient number of well-marked fire exits.
- A well-stocked first-aid box should be clearly visible and accessible.
- Shower and toilet facilities should be available.
- Water and fluids must be kept away from the working area, as spillages make the floor slippery and dangerous.
- There should be no eating or drinking in the working area.
- Exercises should be supervised by qualified instructors at all times.
- Protective mats should be available for floor exercises.
- Mirrors should be available to check body alignment and to correct the performance of activities.

THE CLIENT

- Suitable clothing that will allow free, unrestricted movement must be worn. Cotton is the best fabric, as it allows easy absorption of perspiration. Cotton vests or T-shirts and shorts with elasticated waists, or cotton bodies, are all suitable. Some athletes wear track suits and leg-warmers to maintain or raise body temperature during the warm-up and stretch routines.
- Footwear must be chosen with care to suit the activity. Well-constructed shoes should be bought from a reputable manufacturer. Footwear for exercise should be light and comfortable and offer good lateral support. The toe box should have sufficient height, breadth and length to prevent the toes rubbing. The inner sole should absorb shock and the outer sole should be pliable, durable and non-slip. The tongue should be padded to protect the dorsum of the foot and the heel tab should not be too high and should not press on the heel. Socks alone should never be used for exercise because of the danger of slipping, but they should be worn with shoes to reduce friction.

- Hair should be tied back off the face. Hair combs, slides and pins should be avoided.
- Jewellery should be removed.
- Check for contra-indications: if in doubt, seek a doctor's advice.
- Clients must not exercise after a heavy meal, nor under the influence of alcohol. Allow at least two hours after eating.
- Clients must not exercise if pain-killing drugs have been taken.
- Exercises must be clearly explained to the client and any precautions must be stressed. The client must fully understand the exercise and be aware of potential hazards.
- All equipment to be used must be fully demonstrated, its effect explained and safety factors highlighted.
- Exercise or training must be specific to the individual. Clients must work at their own pace and level, must not exceed their capability and should not be forced or made to compete.
- The different levels of fitness and the age range of those present must always be carefully considered when giving group exercise. Individuals must rest when tired and must not exceed their maximum heart rate.
- Exercises should not cause pain – clients must be advised to stop exercising if pain is experienced.
- Select safe, stable starting positions.
- Ensure that good posture and body alignment are maintained when exercises are performed to prevent stresses and strains.
- Teach the client the correct breathing patterns. They must not hold their breath.
- Ensure that the clients perform a thorough warm-up lasting ten to fifteen minutes that includes all the large muscle groups.
- Ensure that clients stretch carefully, slowly and smoothly, and include all the main joints. After the main activity, make sure that clients perform a cool-down (warm-down). Stretch again, then finish with relaxation and deep breathing.

Remember:

- Do not exercise or stretch cold muscles.
- Always practise warm-up exercises.
- Warming the tissues with various forms of heat therapy and massage will help, but is not enough; warm-up exercises must be done, as they allow the body systems to build up gradually to meet the demand placed on them. Include mobilisers, pulse raisers and simple stretches.
- Increase to peak intensity very gradually and decrease gradually.

Guidelines for exercise

These can be displayed in the exercise room or fully explained to clients at the beginning of the course.

CONSIDERATIONS BEFORE YOU START

- Wear suitable clothing and well-fitting shoes and socks.
- Do not exercise in socks.
- Tie your hair back off the face with ribbons or bands.
- Remove all jewellery except rings.
- Check the list of contra-indications. Do not exercise if you know or suspect that you are affected by any on the list.
- If you are suffering from any other illness, please report it. Check with your doctor whether exercising is suitable.
- Do not exercise after a heavy meal: allow at least two hours to elapse.
- Do not exercise if under the influence of alcohol or pain-killing drugs.
- Do not exercise if you are feeling tired and fatigued, nor if suffering from muscle soreness except delayed onset of muscle soreness following other activities, in which case exercise carefully.
- Empty the bladder before exercise.

CONSIDERATIONS DURING AND AFTER EXERCISE

- Do not strain. Exercise should not produce pain.
- Always work at your own pace. Rest when necessary. Do not compete with others.
- Take your pulse rate at regular intervals and do not exceed the maximum heart rate for your age.
- Keep to a few repetitions at the beginning of the course and add three to five with each session.
- Do not exercise or stretch cold muscles. Always perform a ten to fifteen minute warm-up first. If you are late for the class, do not join in until you have completed the warm-up.
- Learn to perform the exercises correctly. Pay attention to detail.
- Always exercise carefully, paying full attention throughout. Do not exercise half-heartedly, mechanically or without concentration. Movements should be smooth and co-ordinated.

- Stretch carefully, smoothly and slowly, feeling the stretch in the belly of the muscle and not at the tendon ends. Hold the stretch and release slowly.

- Do not bounce at the end of the muscle range or stretch muscles rapidly. This type of ballistic movement works against the stretch reflex and may result in small tears within the muscle.

- Breathe freely during exercise. Do not hold the breath when stretching; exhale as you move into the stretch and effort.

- Maintain good body alignment (posture) while exercising. Avoid strain on vulnerable areas such as the neck, lower back and knees.

- If injury occurs, stop exercising immediately. Follow the 'RICED' principle to deal with injury – rest, ice, compression, elevation and diagnosis.

- Drink water at the end of the session to maintain fluid levels.

Client assessment

The assessment of a client prior to exercise has developed considerably over the last few years. In addition to obtaining information regarding health and medical history and taking measurements of height, weight, fat distribution and muscle tone, it is now desirable to assess fitness by measuring the pulse rate, blood pressure, lung capacity, muscle strength, muscle endurance, flexibility and body composition.

Accurate assessment is important for the following reasons:

- It provides information on the client's past and present state of health. This will highlight any contra-indications or any conditions where caution is necessary.

- It provides information on the client's lifestyle, activities, athleticism and motivation.

- It establishes the figure type, i.e. endomorph, ectomorph or mesomorph. This facilitates the planning and setting of realistic, achievable goals.

- It identifies postural problems and muscle imbalance, so that specific strategies to restore balance can be planned.

- It establishes the current level of fitness, which provides a starting point for the exercise programme.

- It provides the information necessary for setting objectives and planning safe, effective exercise that will not place the client at risk.

- It provides a record of data and the starting point from which future improvement can be measured.

PREPARATION OF THE CLIENT PRIOR TO FITNESS ASSESSMENT

Advise the client:

- to wear comfortable, loose-fitting clothes;
- not to eat for two to three hours before the test;
- not to smoke before or during the test;
- not to drink tea or coffee before the test;
- to empty the bladder before the test;
- to avoid other exercises before the test;
- to concentrate fully on the test;
- to say immediately if they do not understand the instructions and what is required of them.

HEIGHT MEASUREMENT

Method:

- Instruct the client to stand in bare feet with feet together and the back against the measure. Ask the client to stand straight and look directly ahead.
- Bring the measure bar down so that it just touches the head, read the measurement, record it on the client's card and inform the client.

WEIGHT MEASUREMENT

Method:

- Instruct the client to wear minimum clothing (record this to ensure that the same clothing is worn each time the weight is taken), with bare feet. Ask the client to stand still in the centre of the weighing machine and to look directly ahead.
- Read the weight, record it on the client's card and inform the client.

BODY MEASUREMENT

Measurements to be recorded:

- Bust/chest
- Waist

- Hips
- Upper thigh
- Lower thigh
- Upper arms

Method:

- Select a tape measure that is in good condition, not frayed or stretched. Always ensure that the tape is level on the body part and not twisted. Do not pull the tape measure. Use the nearest prominent bony point as a marker. This will ensure that the tape will be placed at the same level each time. Thin elastic can be used to indicate the level.
- Instruct the client to remove all clothing except pants (very self-conscious women may keep a bra on, but they should wear the same bra each time the measurements are taken), stand in bare feet and maintain a good posture, with the arms to the side.

BUST OR CHEST

- Bring the tape around the back, under the armpit and around the nipple line.
- Record the measurement and inform the client.

WAIST

- Give a circle of narrow elastic to the client and ask her to place this at the narrowest part, i.e. her natural waistline. Measure just above the elastic. For males, measure at the level of the navel.
- Record the measurement and inform the client.

HIPS

- Place the tape around the widest part of the hips and measure. Then measure the distance of the tape from the greater trochanter: this will ensure that the tape is placed at the same level next time.
- Record the measurement and inform the client.

RIGHT AND LEFT UPPER THIGH

- Again, use a circle of narrow elastic. Place this around the widest part of the thigh. Measure the distance from the elastic to the top of the patella.
- Place the tape around the leg just above the elastic.
- Record the measurement and inform the client.

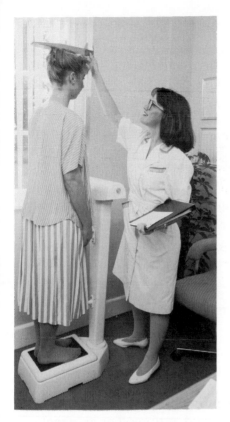

Figure 10.1 *Measuring weight and height*

RIGHT AND LEFT LOWER THIGH

- Use a circle of narrow elastic and place it two to three inches above the top of the patella.
- Place the tape around the leg just above the elastic.
- Record the measurement and inform the client.

RIGHT AND LEFT UPPER ARMS

- Place a circle of narrow elastic around the widest part of the upper arm. Measure the distance from this to the olecranon process.
- Place the tape around the arm just above the elastic.
- Record the measurement and inform the client.

MIDRIFF

- For women whose objective is to lose body weight, measurement of the midriff is necessary. Measure two to three inches below the xiphoid process.

CALF

- For those wishing to build up the calf muscle, measure around the wide part of the calf and note the distance from the tape to the lateral malleolus. Use the same distance next time.

TESTING FOR MUSCLE STRENGTH

Muscle strength is measured by how much weight the muscle is able to move. This is tested using weights or a grip test or by pulling against machines.

WEIGHT LIFT

- Select a suitable stable starting position.
- Select an appropriate weight and check that it is secure.
- Isolate the movement to the muscle being tested.
- Ask the client to lift the weight smoothly to the full inner range three times. If an extra lift is possible, the weight must be increased.
- Ask the client to rest for one to two minutes and repeat the lift with extra weight. The weight that is lifted smoothly two or three times indicates the strength.
- Record the weight.

GRIP TEST

- Make sure the client is holding the grip comfortably in the hand. In the standing position the client lifts the arm above the head, lowers the arm and squeezes as hard as possible. Repeat three times.
- Record the highest reading.

There are a variety of machines on the market designed for testing strength. Read the manufacturer's instructions very carefully, and test a colleague to ensure that you fully understand the procedure.

Exercises such as push-ups and sit-ups are sometimes used to give an indication of fitness, but these are not measurable.

MUSCLE TONE

It is possible to obtain some indication of muscle strength by applying manual resistance to muscle action and feeling the degree of tone within the muscle. This will only provide a rough guide, as it is not possible to quantify the strength but only to categorise it into poor, moderate, good, very good or excellent. Muscles that are easily tested in this way are the biceps and triceps, the abdominals, gluteus maximus and the hip abductors and adductors.

Method:

- Position the client in crook lying. This position can be maintained throughout and avoids moving the client unnecessarily.
- One hand must be placed over the working muscle to feel the tone, while the other hand is used to resist the movement.

BICEPS STRENGTH

- The client bends the elbow to the mid-point of the range.
- Place one hand over the biceps on the anterior aspect of the upper arm. Grasp the wrist with the other.
- Instruct the client to bend the elbow while you stop the movement. Feel the increased tone with the hand placed over the muscle. Is the strength you are feeling poor, moderate, good, very good or excellent? This value judgement becomes easier with practice.
- Record the result.

TRICEPS STRENGTH

- With one hand, cover the triceps on the posterior aspect of the upper arm. Keep the other hand around the wrist.
- Instruct the client to straighten the elbow against resistance. Feel the increased tone with the hand placed over the muscle, and assess the strength.
- Record the result.

ABDOMINAL STRENGTH (PARTICULARLY RECTUS ABDOMINUS)

- Place one hand over the abdominals.
- Instruct the client to perform a curl-up (lifting head and shoulders with chin on chest). If this is done with ease, the free hand can be placed over the sternum and resistance given to the curl-up.
- Feel the increased tone with the hand placed on the abdominals, and assess the strength.
- Record the result.

GLUTEUS MAXIMUS STRENGTH

- Instruct the client to lift his or her bottom up off the bed and tighten the buttocks. (A sandbag weight can be placed over the pelvis to provide resistance.)
- Place a hand over the gluteus maximus.
- Feel the increased tone and judge the strength.
- Record the result.

ABDUCTOR STRENGTH

- Straighten the client's leg.
- Place one hand over the abductors on the outer aspect of the thigh above the greater trochanter.
- Place the other hand under the ankle to cup it.
- Instruct the client to 'push out' towards you. Resist the movement, using the hand at the ankle to push inwards.
- Feel the increased tone in the abductors and judge the strength.
- Record the result.

ADDUCTOR STRENGTH

- Keep the client's leg straight and pulled outwards.
- Keep the hand under the ankle.

- Place the other hand over the adductors on the inner aspect of the thigh (upper third).
- Instruct the client to pull the leg inwards towards the other leg. Resist the movement, using the hand at the ankle to pull outwards.
- Feel the increased tone in the adductors and judge the strength.
- Record the result.

CARDIO-RESPIRATORY ENDURANCE

This may be tested using a treadmill or bicycle ergometer. If this specialised equipment is not available, the step test can be used.

THREE-MINUTE STEP TEST

Equipment:

- Twelve-inch step
- Metronome
- Timing clock/stopwatch
- Stethoscope for measuring heart rate (or take the pulse with the index and middle fingers over the radial artery).

Method:

- Explain the test to the client, demonstrating how to step up and down for three minutes at 24 steps per minute.
- Ask the client to practise.
- Set the metronome to 96 clicks per minute. With each click a foot must move, i.e. click 1: right foot onto step; click 2: left foot onto step; click 3: right foot down off step; click 4: left foot down off step.
- Time the client for three minutes.

Then sit and quickly take the client's pulse or heart rate for one minute. (Count for 30 seconds and multiply by two.) The pulse rate is an excellent indication of cardio-vascular efficiency. If the recorded heart rate is above the maximum heart rate recommended for that client, the client is unfit and must exercise with caution. The client should exercise at a target rate below 50 per cent of MHR. If there is any sign of stress, stop exercising and seek medical advice. As fitness increases and cardio-vascular efficiency increases, the heart rate will decrease. As a rough guide, compare the test result with Table 10.1.

Table 10.1 *The range of heart rates after three minutes' stepping*

	Men aged 20–46	**Women aged 20–46**
Excellent	81–90	79–84
Good	99–102	90–97
Above average	103–112	106–109
Average	120–121	118–119
Below average	123–125	122–124
Fair	127–130	129–134
Poor	136–138	137–145

(Adapted from YMCA *Y's Way to Fitness.*)

Maximum heart rate (MHR)

To calculate Maximum Heart Rate use 220 minus the age of client. Healthy individuals should exercise at a target or training rate of 60–85 per cent of their maximal heart rate. Those at the fair to poor end of the above table would exercise at 60 per cent of the MHR. The fit individuals at the excellent end of the table would need to exercise at the higher end (80–85 per cent) to achieve sufficient overload. See page 96.

Body composition

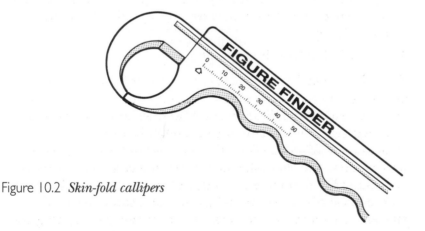

Figure 10.2 *Skin-fold callipers*

Equipment:

- Skin-fold callipers.

Method:

- Identify the locations of the skin folds (see Table 10.2).
- Hold the callipers in the dominant hand.
- Pinch the skin fold with the thumb and forefinger of the other hand.

Table 10.2 *The locations of the skin folds*

Women	Men
Supra-iliac fold diagonally above the crest of the ilium	Abdominal fold vertically 2 cm lateral to umbilicus
Anterior thigh fold vertically midway between knee and hip	Anterior thigh fold vertically midway between knee and hip
Triceps fold vertically midway between elbow and shoulder	Chest fold diagonally halfway between nipple and crease of axilla

- Hold the callipers perpendicular to the skin fold and place the pads very near the thumb and forefinger.
- Close or release the callipers, depending on type.
- Record the measurement.
- Take three or more readings at each skin fold to gain consistency.

The consistent readings at each site are then added together, averaged, and compared with the Table 10.3. This will indicate whether or not there is a need to reduce weight. Measurements may be taken every four to six weeks and compared with previous readings to indicate weight gain or loss. The importance of body composition is explained in full on page 120.

Table 10.3 *The range of body fat percentages*

Women	Men	Rating
less than 25 mm	less than 22 mm	excellent
25 mm–42 mm	22 mm–34 mm	good
43 mm–65 mm	35 mm–73 mm	average
66 mm–82 mm	74 mm–90 mm	fair
over 82 mm	over 90 mm	poor

LUNG CAPACITY MEASUREMENT

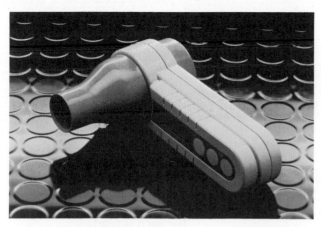

Figure 10.3 *A hand-held spirometer*

Equipment:

- Spirometer and accessories.

Method:

- Ask the client to stand straight, and clip on the nose clip.
- Instruct the client to fill the lungs completely with air with a single deep inhalation, then place the mouth around the disinfected mouthpiece and ensure a perfect seal.
- The client should then breathe out as hard as possible for as long as possible.
- Take three attempts to ensure accurate reading, pausing for three to four minutes between each attempt.
- Read and record the measurements and compare them with charts for normal ranges.

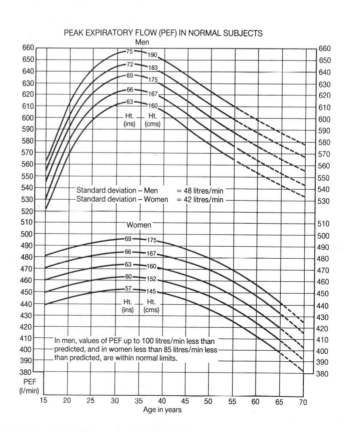

Figure 10.4 *Lung capacities of men and women (I. Gregg, A. J. Nunn,* British Medical Journal, *1973,* **3**, 282)

BLOOD PRESSURE

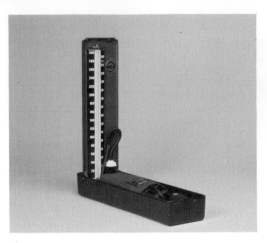

Figure 10.5 *A sphygmomanometer*

Equipment:

- A sphygmomanometer is used to measure blood pressure. The modern models usually found in fitness centres are automatic and give a digital readout. These differ from the models used medically, where a stethoscope is used over the radial artery at the elbow, the sounds during systole and diastole are listened to and the corresponding pressure level for each is read.

Method:

- Normal blood pressure for a young resting adult is about

$$\frac{120 \ \text{(systolic)}}{80 \ \text{(diastolic)}} \ \text{mm Hg}$$ but this varies considerably with activity, emotion and age. Blood pressure tends to rise as we get older. Systolic pressure in adults at rest averages 110–150 mm Hg, diastolic 60–65 mm Hg. *Anyone giving repeated systolic pressure readings of more than of 140 mm Hg should consult a doctor for a check-up before exercising.*

FLEXIBILITY

It is possible to measure lower back and hamstring flexibility for the fit client.

Equipment:

- A box or stool with a tape attached

Method:

- The client should sit with legs stretched out and feet against the box or stool, and with arms stretched forward.
- Ask the client to breathe out, reach forward and slide the hands along the stool. Read the distance at the middle finger. If the box has a slider, the client should push this forward with the hands and the reading is taken.
- Measure for three attempts and record the best result.

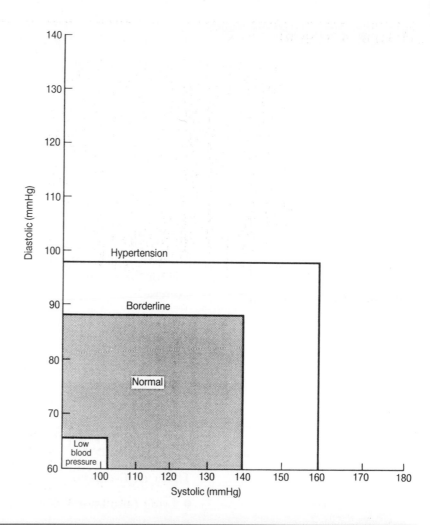

Figure 10.6 *Blood pressure range*

Work with a partner. Practise the different
assessment on each other.

CHAPTER 11

Compiling exercise schemes

When writing out exercise schemes it is vital to state the starting position. This is easily done if schemes are written in two columns: one for the starting position, the other giving instructions for the exercise.

Starting positions

There are five basic starting positions:

- Lying (also known as supine lying)
- Kneeling
- Sitting
- Standing
- Hanging.

These basic positions can be modified to increase or reduce the difficulty of the exercise.

Modifications are made to:

- raise or lower the centre of gravity;
- increase or decrease the size of the base to change stability;
- increase or decrease leverage;
- provide adequate fixation of the body so that specific movements can be performed with maximum concentration;
- increase or decrease the muscle work required to maintain the position;
- ensure maximum support for relaxation.

MODIFICATIONS OF STARTING POSITIONS

- Lying: prone lying, side lying, half lying, crook lying, crook lying with pelvis lifted.

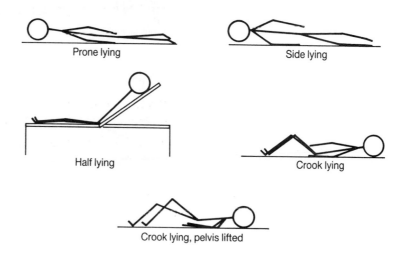

Figure 11.1 *Modifications of lying*

- Kneeling: prone kneeling, inclined prone kneeling, heel sitting, half kneeling.

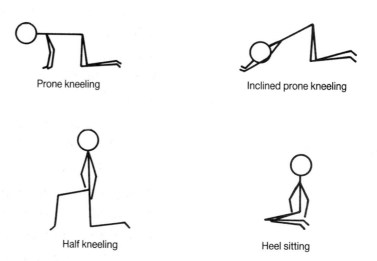

Figure 11.2 *Modifications of kneeling*

- Sitting: crook sitting, long sitting, astride sitting, side sitting, stoop sitting, fall out sitting.

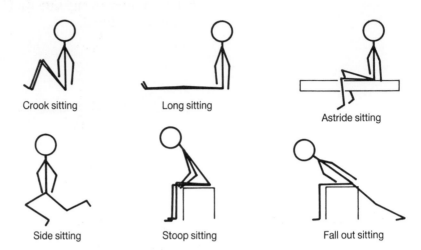

Figure 11.3 *Modifications of sitting*

- Standing: toe standing, stride standing, walk standing, step standing, lax stoop standing, stoop standing.

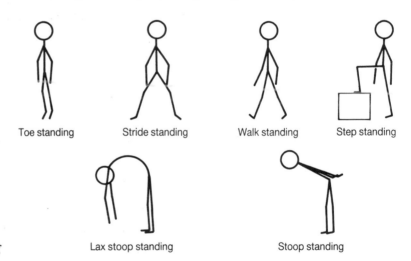

Figure 11.4 *Modifications of standing*

- Hanging: stride hanging, knee bend hanging.

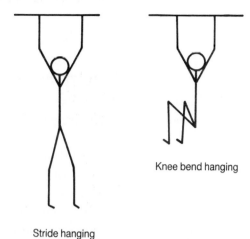

Knee bend hanging

Figure 11.5 *Modifications of hanging*

Stride hanging

The position of the arms is also very important and this is usually written first, e.g. bend stride standing.

- Arm positions: wing, low wing, bend, across bend, under bend, reach, yard, stretch, head rest.

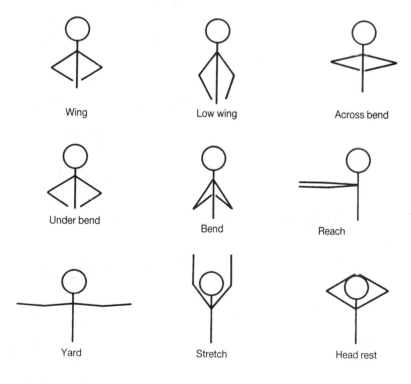

Figure 11.6 *Arm positions*

The progression of exercise

Progression is essential to maintain and improve the beneficial effects of exercise. The work must be progressively increased in order to maintain overload. There are various ways of making exercises more difficult:

- increase the frequency, i.e. the number of times an exercise is performed. Begin with six repetitions, then ten, fifteen and twenty. If muscle endurance is the objective, increase the repetitions to 30–50;
- increase the intensity, i.e. make the muscles work harder by increasing the resistance. Weights, springs, pulley systems, multigyms, etc., are used to provide resistance;
- change the leverage: begin with a short weight arm and increase the length when the work becomes easy. The leg and arm can be shortened by bending the knee and elbow. Progression is achieved by straightening the limb, then holding a pole or dumb-bells. The leverage of curl-ups is increased by moving the arm position from at the side to across the chest, then putting the hands on the shoulders, etc. Leverage and weight can be combined for progression.
- Increase the number of sessions, e.g. from twice to three times per week or more. Ensure that there is sufficient rest time for the body to recover fully, otherwise there is risk of damage.
- To improve cardio-respiratory endurance, increase the duration of the exercise.
- Reduce the stability of the starting position. Exercising becomes more difficult as the starting position becomes less stable. This will improve the skill components of balance, co-ordination and agility.
- Change the speed at which an exercise is performed. Exercises are easier at natural speed, which varies with the individual. Exercises become more difficult if the speed is increased or decreased.

Potentially damaging exercises

There are a number of exercises that produce excessive stress on vulnerable areas of the body, such as the neck, the lower back and the knees, and that may result in injury. Many of these exercises form part of certain training programmes and routines for specific sports. When they are performed by very fit trained athletes in controlled situations the risk of injury is greatly reduced. They should not be performed by unfit individuals, nor included in general exercise or group exercises where individual supervision and control is impossible. The ability to evaluate the safety and effectiveness of an exercise is an important part of an instructor's role. All exercise videos, exercise books and magazine articles should be carefully studied, and each exercise must be analysed and checked for safety, as many of these hazardous exercises are often included. New forms of exercise routines or 'crazes' require particular caution. Because the human body is designed to perform a certain finite number of movements through specific ranges, the so-called 'new' exercises must be versions of the old. Claims made for the results are often exaggerated, and so must be carefully assessed: are they realistic and achievable?

When assessing the safety and effectiveness of an exercise it is useful to ask the following questions:

1 Will the exercise work the appropriate body part?
2 Will the exercise move the selected muscle and joint through the correct range?
3 Will the movement be a controlled, free movement, not forced or ballistic?
4 Is the exercise appropriate for the client's level of fitness?
5 Could the exercise over-stress the moving joints or other body parts, causing damage?
6 Is this the most suitable exercise for achieving the set goal?
7 Will the exercise or the starting position put stress on any of the following vulnerable areas: the cervical region (the neck); the lumbar region (the lower back); the knees?

THE SEVEN VERTEBRAE OF THE CERVICAL REGION

This is the region of greatest spinal mobility. The first two cervical vertebrae – the atlas and axis – allow rotation of the head. The movements of the cervical region are:

- *flexion* – dropping the head forward, chin on chest;
- *extension* – tilting the head backwards – and hyper-extension – taking it beyond extension to look at the ceiling;
- *side flexion* (lateral flexion) – dropping the head sideways, ear towards shoulder;
- *rotation* – turning the head to the right and left, looking towards the shoulder;
- *circumduction* – a combination of the above;

Movements of the chin also affect the cervical region:

- *protraction* of the chin – pushing the chin forward;
- *retraction* of the chin – pulling the chin back and in.

Before commencing exercises for the cervical spine, select a stable starting position such as sitting or stride standing. If the client is very tense, the lying position can be used. Make sure the head is in a good position: erect, with ear lobes level, eyes looking straight ahead and shoulders relaxed.

SAFE EXERCISES

Starting position	Exercise
• Sitting	drop chin onto chest, return to upright position.
• Sitting	take right ear down towards right shoulder and back, then left ear towards left shoulder and back.
• Sitting	turn the head to the right to look towards the right shoulder, repeat to left.

For all these exercises, it is important to keep the chin in and the head up.

NOT RECOMMENDED

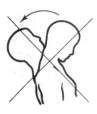

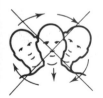

• Sitting	hyper-extension – dropping the head back to look at the ceiling.
• Sitting	circling head around on the shoulders.

The exercises which are not recommended produce excessive pressure on and compression of the cervical discs. These may protrude into the inter-vertebral foramina, resulting in pressure on and damage to the nerves. This will cause pain, numbness and pins and needles over the shoulder and down the arm.

With age the cervical region is susceptible to wear and tear, with erosion of the cartilage and bone. This may result in inflammation of surrounding structures, with pain and stiffness of the neck. These exercises will exacerbate this condition. The movements should only be performed by young, fit well-trained individuals.

They should not be done in general exercise classes, by those over 30 years old or by anyone suffering from headaches, neck pain or shoulder and arm pain, numbness or pins and needles.

NOT RECOMMENDED

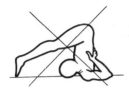

- Lying

lift legs and lower back upwards and touch the floor behind the head with the toes (the 'plough').

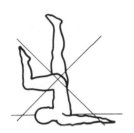

- Lying

lift legs and hips off the floor and support with hands, cycle or open/close legs in the air.

With both these exercises, the body weight is supported across the shoulders and neck. This imposes severe compression forces on the neck, which can cause damage to ligaments, bones, discs and nerves. This position also compresses the chest, thus reducing the working and efficiency of the heart and lungs.

THE FIVE VERTEBRAE OF THE LUMBAR REGION

The lower back is a vulnerable area because it supports the weight of the upper body before it is distributed to the pelvis. The movements of the lumbar region are:

- *flexion* – bending forward;
- *extension* – moving the trunk backwards;
- limited *side flexion* – bending to the side;
- negligible *rotation* – turning the trunk right and left is negligible in the lumbar region; most trunk rotation occurs in the thoracic region.

The lumbar region is where most trunk flexion occurs. It is the fulcrum for this movement, where the weight is the upper trunk and the weight arm is the length of the trunk about the fulcrum. The effort is supplied by the back extensors and the effort arm is the distance of their insertion from the fulcrum.

Considerable stress is placed on the lumbar spine during forward flexion and the return to extension. The amount of stress is influenced by two factors:

1 the length of the weight arm and the amount of weight;
2 the degree of rotation of the pelvis that accompanies the movement.

The trunk extensors (the erector spinae) and the antagonistic trunk flexors (the abdominals) must be strong and balanced to support the trunk and maintain the stability of the pelvis. Imbalance between these muscles alters the pelvic tilt and imposes stresses on the lumbar spine.

- Weakness of the abdominals results in forward pelvic tilt and lordosis of the lumbar spine.

- Weakness of the erector spinae results in backward pelvic tilt and flat back.

SAFE EXERCISE

• Stride standing, hands on legs (knees soft)	slowly bend forwards, sliding the hands down the legs, then return to upright position.

Particular care must be taken when straightening up: always rotate the pelvis backwards first and then extend the lumbar spine. The instruction to clients on returning to the upright position should be to pull their bottom in and straighten inch by inch from the bottom of the spine upwards.

NOT RECOMMENDED

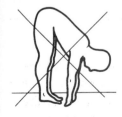

• Stretch, stride standing	bend forward to touch floor and swing up.

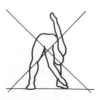

• Stretch, stride standing	bend to touch opposite foot with hand.

In these positions, with the arms stretched above the head, the weight arm is lengthened and there is a far greater load in front of the fulcrum (the lumbar spine). This increases the stress and compression on the discs, and damage can occur to ligaments, discs, cartilage or bones. Punching the air with the hands in forward flexion imposes the same stress and is not recommended. Rotating the trunk to touch the opposite foot increases the compression forces still further.

Ballistic-type bouncing at the end of the range of forward flexion in order to stretch the hamstrings must be avoided. This exerts excessive pressure on the lower back and may produce micro-tears and damage to the hamstrings. Since the hamstrings are not relaxed in this position but are contracting eccentrically, stretching is ineffective and can cause damage.

SAFE EXERCISE	• Stride standing	trunk side flexion to the right and left.

The same principle of leverage applies to this exercise, which will be safe if the arms are kept down to the side, keeping the weight arm as short as possible.

NOT RECOMMENDED	• Stride standing	swing left arm into the air and side flex laterally to the right, then return and swing right arm up and side flex laterally to the left.

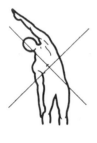

The arm is stretched up into the air, increasing the length of the weight arm. The increased leverage imposes stresses on the lumbar joints and discs, causing damage. Again, ballistic bouncing at the end of the range will make the exercise even more hazardous.

NOT RECOMMENDED	• Side lying	lift both legs upwards.

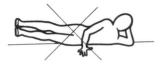

The trunk side flexors will strain to lift the legs. This stresses the lower back. Twisting of the trunk while straining to lift the legs causes further damage.

ABDOMINAL STRENGTHENING EXERCISES

SAFE EXERCISES

• Crook lying	press small of back into floor, tilt pelvis backwards and pull in the abdominals.
• Crook lying, hands across chest	curl up head towards knees.

The second exercise can be safely progressed by moving the arm position, thus lengthening the weight arm: for example with the hands on the shoulders, the hands beside the head, the hands stretched above the head. (The hands should not, however, be clasped behind the head, as this can stress and damage the neck; instead, place the hands beside the head above the ears.)

The exercise can be progressed further by holding a weight across the chest and above the head.

NOT RECOMMENDED

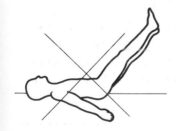

• Lying	double leg raising.
• Lying	straight leg sit-ups.

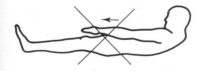

Both these exercises impose stress and can cause many problems. They are not effective in strengthening the abdominal muscles, as can be seen by analysing the movement:

Moving joint:	hip joint
Direction of movement:	flexion coming up, extension going down
Prime movers:	psoas (hip flexor)
Muscle work:	concentric coming up, eccentric going down.

The psoas is a short muscle passing from the lumbar vertebrae to the lesser trochanter of the femur. It works with the iliacus and both muscles may be named ilio-psoas. As the psoas lifts the legs or the trunk it pulls on its origin on the lumbar spine, imposing stresses and strains in this region. The psoas is working at tremendous mechanical disadvantage, as it is made to lift a long weight arm with a large weight (that of the legs). The back arches and strain is felt in the lumbar spine.

With this exercise, the psoas becomes stronger and tighter. This is undesirable, because a tight psoas pulls and tilts the pelvis forwards, resulting in lordosis due to muscle imbalance.

The abdominal muscles will be working statically in outer range in an attempt to keep the pelvis level. This type of muscle work is extremely difficult to maintain and can only be done by very strong muscles; weaker muscles will be strained.

Static work of the abdominals increases intra-abdominal pressure, which will push on the pelvic organs and stretch the pelvic floor. The muscles of the pelvic floor may already be weakened in post-natal women and older age groups. Strength must be maintained in the pelvic floor to prevent incontinence.

BACK STRENGTHENING EXERCISES

SAFE EXERCISES

• Prone lying	alternate single leg raising.
• Prone lying	alternate arm raising.
• Prone lying	opposite arm and leg raising.

NOT RECOMMENDED

- Prone lying   double leg raising.

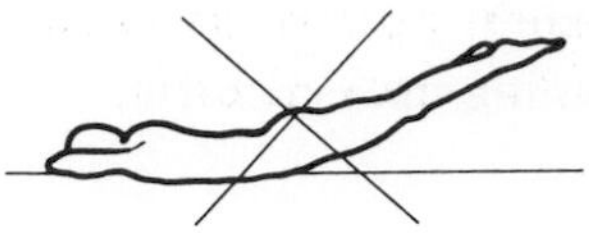

- Prone lying   double leg, arm and trunk raising.

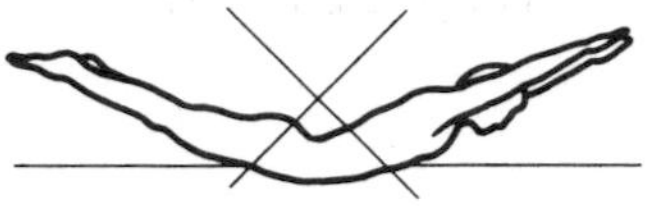

- Prone lying   trunk extension, touching feet with hands.

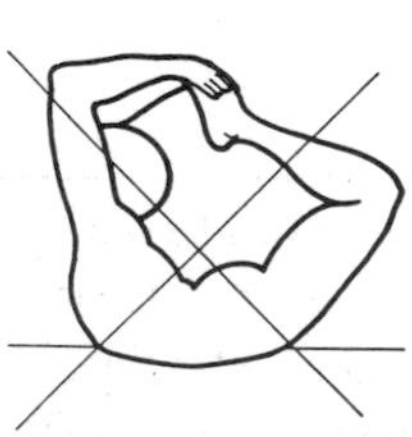

Raising both legs or, worse, raising both legs and arms, imposes severe compression and stress on the lumbar spine.

GLUTEAL STRENGTHENING EXERCISES

SAFE EXERCISES

- Prone lying   raise alternate legs off the floor and lower (keep hips in contact with the floor and raise legs only fifteen degrees from floor).
- Prone kneeling   straighten alternate legs backwards (lifting no more than fifteen degrees from horizontal) and lower.

NOT RECOMMENDED

- Prone kneeling   bend knee onto chest and kick out behind.

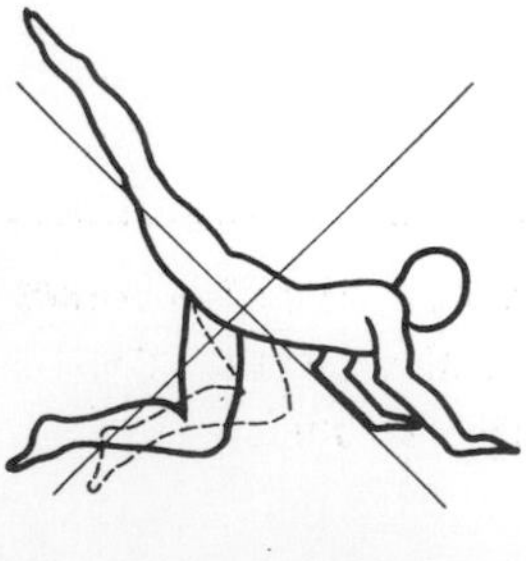

Raising the leg more than fifteen degrees above the horizontal can stress the lumbar spine. Also, this exercise uses the hip flexor (iliopsoas) to bend the knee towards the chest (this does not usually require strengthening). This exercise is frequently performed in a swinging manner, where the movement is not controlled and is likely to cause damage.

THE KNEE JOINT

The stability of the knee is maintained by several strong ligaments (the medial and lateral ligaments and the cruciate ligaments), by powerful muscles (the quadriceps and hamstrings) and by the fascia of the thigh (the fascia lata).

The movements of the knee are:

- *flexion* – bending the knee;
- *extension* – straightening the knee;
- a slight amount of *rotation* in flexion.

SAFE EXERCISE		
	• Long sitting	bend right knee and rotate hip outwards, drop knee onto floor and place foot against left thigh. Place hands on either side of left leg and gently slide hands down left leg forwards. Repeat on opposite side.

NOT RECOMMENDED

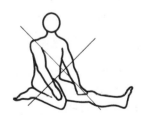

	• Long sitting	bend right knee, turn leg backwards, slide hands along left leg to touch toes (hurdler's stretch).

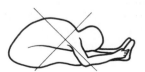

	• Long sitting	forward flexion, bringing head down onto knees.

The flexion of the knee backwards in the hurdler's stretch stresses the medial ligaments of the knee. This method also stresses the lower back, as excessive forward flexion stresses the back.

NOT RECOMMENDED

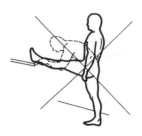

•	Standing	right leg propped up at right angles, bend forwards sliding hands down left leg.

SAFE EXERCISE

•	Standing, stride or walk standing	bend knees until they are at 90°, bend. Do not allow buttocks to go below the knees.

NOT RECOMMENDED

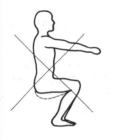

•	Standing, stride or walk standing	bend or squat beyond 90°, allowing the buttocks to go below the knees.

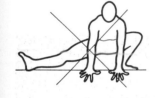

•	Standing	squatting then jumping and stretching leg out to side.

Squatting and bending the knees beyond 90° while they are supporting the body weight can impose severe stress on the knee joint.

NOT RECOMMENDED

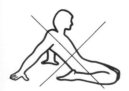

'Heel sitting' should be avoided by all except the young and very fit, as it stresses and can damage the knee joint. In this position the weight of the body pulls the knee joint open, and this can damage the cartilage and strain the ligaments.

Kneeling and modifications of kneeling should not be used as a starting position for the older client, nor for anyone with knee pain.

DAMAGING EXERCISES THAT SHOULD BE AVOIDED

- Double leg raising or sit-ups with straight legs
- Hurdler's stretch, either standing or long sitting
- Pliés
- Deep squats
- Forward flexion where the trunk is at 90° to the legs
- The 'plough' (resting on head and shoulders with the legs in the air)
- Head circling
- Head hyper-extension
- Very wide 'jumping jacks' with the knees opening wider than the toes: keep the knees in line with the toes
- Any ballistics, i.e. bouncing at the end of range in stretches such as toe touching, side bending, trunk twisting
- Moving from heel sitting up to kneeling, except for the young and athletic (i.e. those with strong quadriceps). It should not be performed by anyone with knee problems nor those over 50. The same applies to exercises using kneeling as a starting position
- Back hyper-extension.

T A S K S

Work with a partner.

- Teach your partner safe head and neck movements.
- Teach your partner safe trunk forward flexion, side flexion and back extension exercises.
- Explain why the following movements should not be performed:

a head circling and hyper-extension

b double leg raising and straight leg sit-ups

c deep squatting with the bottom lower than the knees.

CHAPTER 12

General exercises

Warm-up exercises

These exercises are performed at the beginning of an exercise class or athletic performance. They bring the body slowly to a level that will enable the individual to perform at maximal potential and will also reduce the risk of injury. The length of time spent on the warm-up will depend on environmental temperature. On cold days a longer warm-up will be required. The warm-up should be long enough to produce light sweating. This is a good indication that the body temperature has been raised sufficiently to begin the stretch programme. A warm-up should be performed for fifteen to twenty minutes. Exercises should increase in intensity very gradually and decrease gradually. They must include mobilising exercises and pulse raisers before the stretch.

The warm-up

- raises body temperature;
- increases cardio-respiratory response;
- increases blood flow to the muscles, and thus increases oxygen and nutrient delivery
- increases muscle cellular metabolism;
- increases the speed of nerve impulse transmission to the muscles;
- increases muscle elasticity and extensibility, thus reducing stiffness and the risk of tear injuries;
- raises hormonal response.

All the large muscle groups must be included in the warm-up, namely the muscles of the calf, the quadriceps, the hamstrings, the abdominals and the shoulder muscles. It is also important to include all the muscles used in the main exercise scheme or athletic performance. These may include the hip abductors and adductors, gluteus maximus, pectorals, trapezius, back extensors, biceps and triceps.

Always begin with easy, gentle exercises, progress to the more difficult and then end with gentle exercises.

EXAMPLES OF WARM-UP EXERCISES

Warm-up exercises may be selected from the following:

- Alternate heel raising
- Stepping, step-kicks
- Walking around the room
- Brisk walking around the room
- Marching on the spot
- Marching around the room
- Knee bend and grasp with hands
- Skipping
- Jumping jacks (caution: do not abduct too far)
- Alternate leg swinging forwards and backwards
- Alternate leg swinging sideways
- Hip circling
- Pelvic tilting forwards and backwards
- Hip and trunk rotation clockwise and anti-clockwise
- Trunk twisting to right and left
- Trunk side bends (caution: keep arms to sides)
- Shoulder shrugging
- Shoulder circling backwards and forwards
- Arm swinging across body, chest press, shoulder press
- Arm circling, beginning with small circles and increasing the range, or upward rowing
- Elbow bending and extending with backward arm swing
- Alternate arm and trunk upward stretch
- Neck flexion, extension, side flexion and rotation
- Combine leg and arm movements

Cool-down exercises

These exercises are performed for ten to fifteen minutes at the end of the class. They allow the body to return slowly to a state of balance (homeostasis). The steady pumping action of muscle contraction keeps the blood flowing through the muscles, thus removing waste products such as lactic acid, which would cause pain and stiffness. The cool-down should include some stretching exercises for the main muscle groups to reduce soreness.

Do not stand still when performing the cool-down: walk, jog or perform the exercises in a sitting or lying position. This is because the large blood vessels supplying the muscles of the legs are still dilated to meet the demand for more blood while exercising and the peripheral vessels are dilated to lose heat. While the leg muscles are contracting they pump the blood back to the heart, but when standing still these muscles are not pumping and blood pools in the dilated blood vessels due to the pull of gravity. The heart is unable to maintain a sufficient blood supply to the brain, resulting in dizziness and fainting.

EXAMPLES OF COOL-DOWN EXERCISES

- Skipping
- Jogging
- Walking
- Stepping
- Knee bends to chest

In sitting:

- Neck flexion, extension, side flexion, rotation
- Shoulder shrugging
- Trunk rotation
- Trunk side flexion
- Trunk forward flexion
- Alternate knee bending, grasp with hands and pull
- Latissimus dorsi and triceps stretch

In lying:

- Spinal rotation stretch
- Knee-hug hamstring stretch
- Shoulder rotations
- Gastrocnemius stretch

In prone lying:

- Push-up back extension
- Knee-bend quadriceps stretch

In long sitting

- Gastrocnemius stretch

- Hamstring stretch
- Spinal rotation stretch

Descriptions of these exercises are found on pages 189–201.

End the class with deep breathing in the lying position and get up slowly.

Strengthening exercises

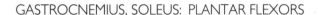

CALF STRENGTHENING EXERCISES

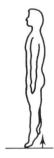

GASTROCNEMIUS, SOLEUS: PLANTAR FLEXORS

Starting position	*Exercise*
• Standing	lift up onto toes and down.
• Standing on one leg	lift up onto toes and down. Repeat with other leg.
• Standing	step onto a step, then lift onto toes. Repeat with other leg.

When these three exercises become too easy and the client can perform 20–30 without difficulty, weights can be used to increase the effort. Hold equal weights in each hand, beginning with 1 kg and increasing gradually as muscle strength improves.

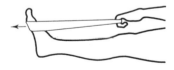

• Long sitting with resistance rubber belt around the feet held by hands	push both feet against the belt, then push alternate feet against the belt.
or	use multigym and plantar flex against the resistance.

The following activities will also improve the strength and mobility of the foot and ankle:

- Walking: push off onto toes
- Jumping: pushing from toes
- Hop on one foot and then the other
- Skip on the toes

- Sprint from one wall to another
- Run or jog on a flat surface
- Run or jog up a hill
- Jump across a bench, either with bunny jumps or straight.

QUADRICEPS STRENGTHENING EXERCISES

RECTUS FEMORIS, VASTUS MEDIALIS, VASTUS LATERALIS, VASTUS INTERMEDIUS: KNEE EXTENSORS

Starting position	*Exercise*
• Long sitting	press the back of the knee down into the bed and tighten the quadriceps muscle: dorsi-flex the foot and try to lift the heel just off the bed. Hold and release.
• Long sitting with a rolled towel under the heel	press the back of the knee downwards and tighten the quadriceps muscle; dorsi-flex the foot. Hold and release.
• Long sitting	dorsi-flex the foot and tighten the knee. Raise the leg just off the bed, keeping the knee tight and straight.

If the knee bends slightly it indicates that the muscle is weak and that the above exercises must be continued until the leg can be lifted without any give.

• Long sitting	dorsi-flex the foot and tighten the knee, then lift the leg and circle it slowly around.

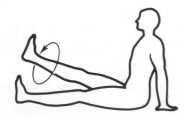

- Long sitting

dorsi-flex the foot and tighten the knee, lift the leg and lower it almost to the bed, then lift it again several times.

- Long sitting

dorsi-flex the foot and tighten the knee, lift the leg and swing it out sideways. Repeat several times.

- Long sitting with tightly rolled towel behind knee under thigh

dorsi-flex the foot and lift the lower leg to straighten the knee, then lower.

- Crook sitting

straighten alternate legs, keeping thighs parallel.

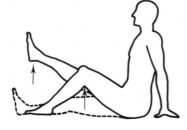

- Long sitting with a weight across the ankle

dorsi-flex the foot, keeping the heel clear of the ground as the knee is tightened. Then lift the leg and weight off the bed. Hold and lower. (Do not lift too high – 24 cm is enough.) Begin with a weight that can just be lifted with a straight knee.

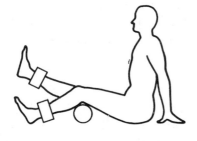

- Long sitting with rolled towel behind the knee, weight over ankle as above

press the back of the knee into the towel and straighten the knee. Hold and release.

- High sitting on a high chair or on the edge of a couch, feet off the floor and knee at 90°. Weight strapped to ankle as above.

Slowly lift the weight until the knee is straight. Keep the thigh in contact with the couch. Hold and lower slowly back to 90° bend. Repeat ten times, then rest for one minute. Repeat again until weight is lifted 30 times. Then increase weight. If the knee cannot fully straighten, the weight is too great. Repeat with a lower weight.

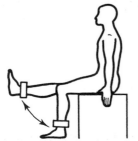

This last exercise can be performed with an elasticated band or spring attached to the chair, level with the ankle, against which the leg then pulls. Use a leg-press machine if available.

Note: before using weights to improve strength, read the notes on weight training in chapter 8.

• Wing standing	bend the knees and lower the body slowly, bending to just above a right angle. Keep the back straight. Push up straight and lock the knees by pulling patella upwards. (Caution: do not take the buttocks below knee level.)

This can be progressed by holding a weight in the arms or by placing them over the shoulders. A fit person could perform this with one leg at a time.

• Using a multigym or sliding sprung board or rowing machine	bend the knees fully. Then push out to straighten and tighten the knees, hold it and bend the knees again slowly. Keep the back straight.
• Standing in front of a bench or stairs	step up, straighten the knee fully, then step down. Do ten or more per leg. A fit person could step up and down two stairs at a time.

Cycling is also beneficial to the quadriceps muscle. Make sure that the leg can straighten during each downward movement of the pedal. To progress, increase the resistance as necessary on an exercise bike or cycle uphill on an ordinary bicycle.

Hamstring strengthening exercises

BICEPS FEMORIS, SEMIMEMBRANOSUS, SEMITENDINOSUS: KNEE
FLEXORS AND HIP EXTENSORS

Starting position	*Exercise*
• High sitting, heel resting on floor	press alternate heels into the floor.
• High sitting with heels against the chair legs	press the back of the heel alternately into the chair legs. Progress by sitting forward so that the knee is bent to a greater angle.
• Standing	bend alternate knees to a right angle and extend the hip (push it backwards).
• Standing with weight around ankles	bend alternate knees to a right angle and extend the hip. Progress by extending with a straight leg.
• Prone lying	cross the legs at the ankles, bend the leg underneath and resist with leg on top.
• Prone lying with weights around ankle	bend alternate knees to a right angle and lift the leg upwards from the hip.
• Prone lying with bent knees, with an elastic strap or spring tied to the ankle and behind at ankle level, or use a multigym	bend the knee to a right angle against the resistance.

HIP EXTENSOR STRENGTHENING EXERCISES

GLUTEUS MAXIMUS: HIP EXTENSOR

Starting position	Exercise
• Supine lying or high sitting	tighten buttocks, then release.
• Supine lying	tighten buttocks and lift slightly off the floor.
• Crook lying	lift buttocks off the floor.
• Standing	swing alternate legs forwards and backwards, lowering slowly.
• Stride standing	slide arms down the legs, bend trunk forwards and return to upright.
• Standing with weights on ankles	swing alternate legs backwards and lower slowly.
• Standing with weights on ankles	bend the knee to a right angle and press the leg backwards with short movements.
• High sitting	stand up and sit down slowly.
• High sitting	press the thighs downwards into the seat and rotate them outwards.
• Prone lying	bend alternate knees and lift the leg off the floor. (Caution: keep the hips against the floor.) Ankle weights can be used for progression.

• Prone lying	lift alternate legs off the floor. (Caution: keep the hips against the floor.)
• Prone kneeling	lift leg backwards and upwards (ankle weights can be used for progression).
• Prone lying with weights around ankle	lift alternate legs off the floor.
• Stoop standing with trunk supported on the bed	raise alternate legs backwards and upwards. Keep the knee straight and the hips on the bed. Ankle weights can be used for progression.
• Prone lying on couch with one leg over the edge	lift the hanging leg backwards and upwards. Repeat with the other leg. Repeat with weights around the ankles.

ABDUCTOR STRENGTHENING EXERCISES

GLUTUS MEDIUS, GLUTEUS MINIMUS AND TENSOR FASCIA LATA: HIP ABDUCTORS AND MEDIAL ROTATORS

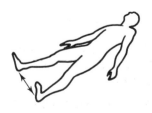

Starting position	*Exercise*
• Supine lying	part the legs and then close them.
• Supine lying	lift alternate legs slightly, move them out to the side and return to the centre.
• High sitting or lying with feet inside the legs of a chair	push both legs outwards against the legs of the chair, hold, then release.
• As above	use a partner and push against his or her legs.

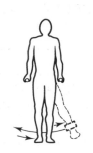

- Support standing

keeping the back straight, swing alternate legs slowly out sideways and back. Occasionally hold the leg in abduction.

- Support standing with weights on ankles

as above, swing alternate legs slowly out sideways and back. Hold in abduction.

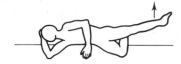

- Side lying with underneath leg bent for balance

lift the upper leg, hold and lower. Keep the hip pushed forwards throughout. Progress using weights.

Note: when this last exercise is performed correctly only 35–40° of abduction is possible, due to the structure of the joint. Individuals may gain greater range by rolling the hip backwards, but this brings the hip flexors into play and therefore does not work the abductors.

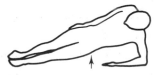

- Side lying with weight on elbow

push the pelvis upwards to arch away from the floor.

ADDUCTOR STRENGTHENING EXERCISES

ADDUCTOR MAGNUS, ADDUCTOR LONGUS, ADDUCTOR BREVIS, PECTINEUS AND GRACILIS: HIP ADDUCTORS AND LATERAL ROTATORS

Starting position	Exercise
• Supine lying	part the legs and then close them.
• Supine lying	lift alternate legs slightly, move them out to the side and then back across the other leg.
• Supine lying	bend the knees onto the chest and then straighten the legs into the air, keeping them at 90°. Scissor the legs open and across.
• High sitting or lying with feet outside the legs of a chair	push both legs inwards against the legs of the chair, hold and release.
• As above	use a partner and push against his or her legs.
• Crook lying	part the knees and then close them. Repeat with the hands on the inside of the knees, pushing against the movement.
• Crook lying	place a pillow or firm sponge between the knees and press the knees together.
• Support standing	keeping the back straight, swing alternate legs out slowly sideways and return across the other leg, hold and release.
• Support standing with weights on ankles	as above, swing alternate legs out slowly sideways and return slowly across the other leg, hold and release.
• Side lying with upper leg bent	raise lower leg upwards, hold and release. Progress by using heavier weights.

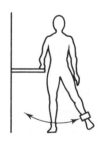

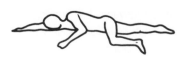

ABDOMINAL STRENGTHENING EXERCISES

RECTUS ABDOMINUS, EXTERNAL OBLIQUE, INTERNAL OBLIQUE,
TRANSVERSUS ABDOMINUS: TRUNK FLEXORS, SIDE FLEXORS
AND ROTATORS

Starting position	*Exercise*
• Crook lying	press the small of the back into the floor, tilt the pelvis backwards and pull the stomach in. Hold and release.
• Crook lying	press the small of the back into the floor. Tuck the head down onto the chest, then raise the head and shoulders to look at the knees. Hold and release.
• Crook lying	bring both knees up to form right angles at hip and knee. Reach up towards the ceiling with alternate knees.
• Crook lying, arms at side	curl up to the knees. (Caution: return slowly from the base of the spine upwards.)
• Crook lying, arms across chest	curl up to the knees.
• Crook lying, hands on shoulders	curl up to the knees.
• Crook lying, hands on ears	curl up towards the knees. (Do not put the hands behind the neck as this can damage the neck.)
• Stretch crook lying	curl up towards the knees. (Caution: only for those with strong abdominals.) Keep the arms back: do not swing them forwards.
• Crook lying, holding a weight or medicine ball on the chest	curl up towards the knees. (Caution: only for those with strong abdominals.)
• Crook lying, holding a weight or medicine ball above the head	curl up towards the knees. (Caution: only for those with strong abdominals.)

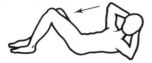

- Crook lying, hands on shoulders

  twist to turn the right elbow towards the left knee, return and repeat with the opposite side.

- Reach crook lying

  curl up and take both the arms to the outside of the left leg, return and repeat on the other side.

- Crook lying

  bend the knees onto the chest and then stretch the legs towards the ceiling. Reach upwards to the ceiling with the feet.

- Crook lying

  bend the knees onto the chest and then stretch the legs towards the ceiling. Keeping the feet together make small circles in the air.

BACK STRENGTHENING EXERCISES

ERECTOR SPINAE, QUADRATUS LUMBORUM: BACK EXTENSORS AND SIDE FLEXORS

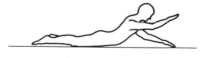

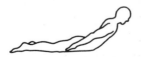

Starting position	*Exercise*
• Prone lying	lift alternate legs and lower.
• Stretch prone lying	lift alternate arms and lower.
• Stretch prone lying	stretch the left arm and right leg along the floor, then lift them slightly and release. Repeat with the other arm and leg.
• Prone lying, arms to sides	keeping the chin in to the chest, lift the head and shoulders, then lower slowly.
• Prone lying, hands clasped behind back	keeping the chin in and the elbows straight, lift the head and shoulders, then lower them slowly.

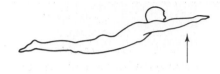

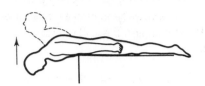

• Stretch prone lying	keeping the chin in, lift the arms, head and shoulders, then lower them slowly. This may be progressed by holding weights in the hands.
• Prone lying, arms to side, with the head and shoulders over the edge of the bed (fix the feet)	lift the head and shoulders as high as possible, then slowly lower them.
• As above with hands on shoulders	lift the arms, head and shoulders as high as possible, then slowly lower them.

Note: these exercises should not be undertaken by anyone with back problems or pain.

TRAPEZIUS AND RHOMBOID STRENGTHENING EXERCISES

RETRACTORS OF THE SHOULDER GIRDLE

Starting position	*Exercise*
• Stride standing	circle the shoulders backwards alternately and then together.
• Stride standing	pull the shoulders down and backwards.
• Across bend stride standing	pull the elbows backwards and release, then straighten the arms and pull backwards.

This last exercise, commonly called 'pull pull fling', should be done slowly and deliberately, as too fast a movement activates the stretch reflex within the muscle and may result in micro-tears of the myofibrils (see chapter 8).

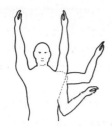

• Standing with heels 10cm away from wall	flatten the back against the wall and stretch the arms above the head, palms facing forward. Keeping the back against the wall, slide the arms down along the wall, bending the elbows. Slide the arms up and down the wall.

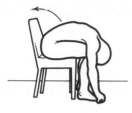

• High sitting, hands on thighs	bend forward with the chest to the thighs. Raise the trunk inch by inch, pushing shoulders into the back of the chair.
• High sitting	bend forward as above, but raise the trunk against the resistance of a therapist applying force behind the shoulders.
• Prone lying	keeping the chin in, raise the head and shoulders off the floor, hold and release, then lower slowly.
• Prone lying, hands clasped behind back	keeping the chin in, pull the shoulders back and lift the head and shoulders off the floor. Hold and lower slowly.
• Prone lying, hands on shoulders	keeping the chin in, pull the shoulders back and lift the head and shoulders off the floor. Hold and lower slowly.
• Yard prone lying	keeping the chin in, lift the arms backwards and raise the head and shoulders off the floor.

SERRATUS ANTERIOR AND TRICEPS STRENGTHENING EXERCISES

POSITIONING OF SCAPULA DURING MOVEMENTS OF THE ARM AND HOLDING THE SCAPULA AGAINST THE CHEST WALL. THE SAME EXERCISES ARE USED FOR THE EXTENSOR OF THE ELBOW TRICEPS

Starting position	Exercise
• Across bend stride standing	pull the elbows back and straighten the arms out to the side slowly and deliberately.
• Bend stride standing	punch the air, a pillow, a punch bag or the therapist's hands.
• Bend stride standing	push forwards against the resistance of the therapist, first with both hands, then alternately.
• Bend stride standing	straighten the arms up above the head alternately and then together.
• Stride standing or high sitting	lean the body forwards, straighten the arms and stretch them backwards. (Hand weights can be used for progression.)
• Stride standing, arms bent, hands on wall	push the body away from the wall by straightening the elbows.
• Prone kneeling	bend and straighten the elbows.
• Prone lying	bend and straighten the elbows, lifting the upper trunk (half press-up).
• Prone lying	press-up.
• Crook lying, holding weights in hands at shoulder level	push the weights vertically upwards and lower them, first alternately, then together. Progress by increasing the weights.

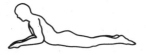

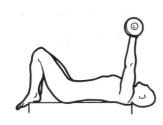

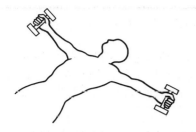

- Yard crook lying

holding the weights, raise the arms from the side to ceiling. Progress by increasing the weights.

These exercises should not be performed by a client with round shoulders as they strengthen the pectoral muscles.

Stretching exercises

STRETCHING THE FOOT

Starting position	Exercise
• Sitting, legs crossed at knee	gently and evenly pull the toes upwards and then the foot. Hold and relax.
• Sitting, legs crossed at knee	gently and evenly push the foot downwards and then the toes. Hold and relax.
• Heel sitting	with bare feet, sit back on the heels and feel the pull on the top of the foot. Hold and relax. (Caution: not to be performed by anyone with knee problems.)
• Standing	place the toes vertically against a step, rock forwards and raise the heels off the ground.

CALF STRETCHING

GASTROCNEMIUS AND SOLEUS

Starting position	*Exercise*
• Long sitting, back against wall	keep the knees straight and strongly dorsi-flex the feet (do not invert or evert). Hold for a count of ten and release. (A strap can be placed around the balls of the feet and pulled towards the body for additional stretch.)
• Walk standing, one foot directly in front of the other	keep the back heel firmly on the ground and bend the front knee gently until a pull is felt in the calf of the hind leg. Hold for a count of ten, then slowly release. Repeat with the other leg.
• Reach standing, facing a wall, with hands against wall	walk the feet backwards, keeping the heels on the ground, until a pull is felt in the calves. Hold for a count of ten.
• Standing with hands against wall as above	walk the feet backwards, keeping the heels on the ground. When the pull is just being felt, bend the elbows slowly and the pull will increase. Hold for a count of ten.
• Standing on an incline	lean forward, keeping the heels on the ground, until a pull is felt in the calf.
• Toe standing on the edge of a step	lift up onto the toes and align the body over the feet, then lower the heels until the pull is felt in the calf. Hold for a count of ten, then release.
• Reach standing, hands against wall	keeping the heels on the ground, bend both knees, then take the body forward over the feet until the pull is felt in the calf. Hold for a count of ten, then release.

Front of thigh stretching

QUADRICEPS GROUP: RECTUS FEMORIS, VASTUS MEDIALIS, VASTUS LATERALIS AND VASTUS INTERMEDIUS

Starting position	*Exercise*
• Support standing	standing on one leg, grasp the other leg from behind around the ankle. Pull the leg backwards until the pull is felt in the front of the thigh. Hold for a count of ten, then release. Keep the trunk straight and avoid rotating the hip and knee outwards. Repeat with the other leg.
• Prone lying	bend the right knee towards the buttock, grasp the ankle and pull until the pull is felt in the front of the thigh. Hold for a count of ten, then release. Keep the front of the hip joint against the floor. Repeat with the other leg.

Fit individuals with no back problems can repeat the the above exercise with both knees bent, pulling on both ankles together.

• Side lying	bending one leg, pull the heel towards the buttocks. Repeat with the other leg.
• Kneeling	lean backwards, keeping the hips pushed forward, until a pull is felt in front of thigh. Hold for a count of ten, then sit forward. (Caution: not for older clients or anyone with knee problems.)
• Kneeling	lean backwards, supporting the weight on the hands behind the body, and push the hips forward. Hold for a count of ten and release. (Caution: not to be performed by older clients or anyone with knee problems.)

Young fit individuals may repeat this last exercise using elbow support behind.

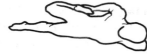

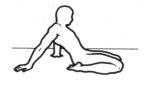

BACK OF THIGH STRETCHING

HAMSTRINGS: BICEPS FEMORIS, SEMIMEMBRANOSUS, SEMITENDINOSUS

Starting position	Exercise
• Supine lying with hips and knees at right angles and feet against a wall	slide the right leg up the wall, dorsi-flex the foot and tighten the knee. Keeping the leg straight and the bottom on the floor, lift the leg away from the wall. Hold for a count of ten and place the foot back on the wall. Repeat with the other leg.
• Crook lying	lift the right leg up and clasp the hands behind the knee. Straighten the knee and dorsi-flex the foot until the pull is felt in the back of the thigh. Hold for a count of ten and lower back to crook. Repeat with the other leg. (Caution: stop if the back arches.)
• Standing in front of a stool or stairs	place one leg onto the stool or the second step of the stairs. Reach forward towards the foot, keeping the back straight and the head in line. Move forward until the pull is felt in the back of the thigh. Hold for a count of ten and release. Repeat with the other leg.
• Sitting with one leg extended on a plinth	straighten the back and lower the trunk onto the thigh. Repeat with the other leg.
• Hurdler's stretch	bend other leg and place foot against inner thigh. Roll knees out slightly. With straight back and head in line, lean over straight leg until pull is felt in back of the thigh.

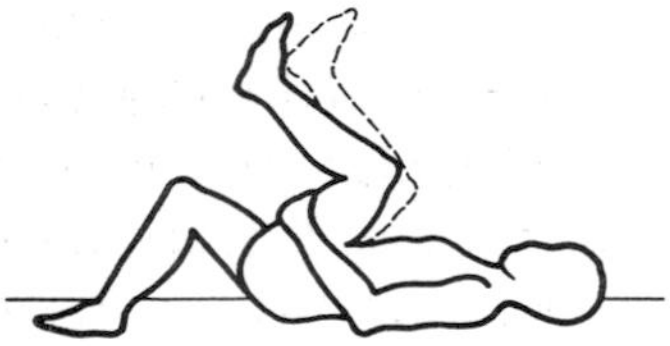

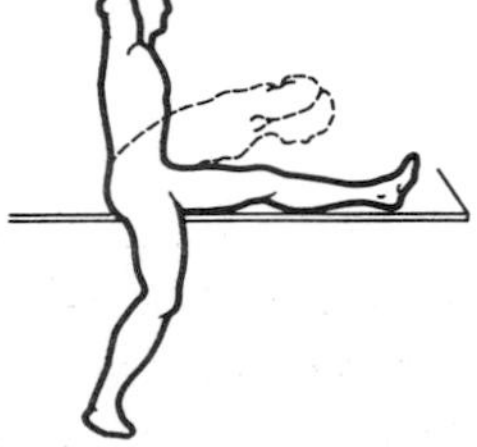

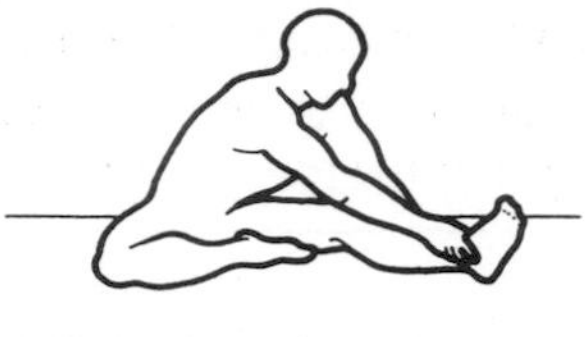

Figure 12.52 *Hurdler's stretch – sitting with one leg extended*

INNER THIGH STRETCHING

ADDUCTOR GROUP: ADDUCTOR LONGUS, ADDUCTOR MAGNUS, ADDUCTOR BREVIS, PECTINEUS, GRACILIS

Starting position	Exercise
• Long sitting	open the legs as far as possible. Keep the back straight and lean forwards until a pull is felt in the inner thigh. Hold for a count of ten and release. (Caution: do not round the trunk or slouch.)
• Crook sitting	keep the feet together and drop the knees open as far as possible. Then pull the feet towards the body until the pull is felt in the inner thigh. Hold for a count of ten and release. (Caution: not to be done by anyone with knee or hip problems.)
• Crook lying, hands on knees	part the knees as far as possible, then press apart with the hands until the pull is felt on the inside of the thigh. Hold for a count of ten and release. (Caution: not to be done by anyone with knee or hip problems.)
• Supine lying, legs up against a wall	part the legs by sliding them along the wall until a stretch is felt in the inner thigh. Hold for a count of ten and release.
• Stride standing	stretch the right leg out as far sideways as possible, without rotating the leg outwards, then bend the left leg until a pull is felt on inner thigh of the right leg. Hold for a count of ten and release. Repeat with the other leg.

OUTER THIGH STRETCHING

HIP ABDUCTORS: GLUTEUS MEDIUS, GLUTEUS MINIMUS, TENSOR FASCIA LATA

Starting position	Exercise
• Supine lying	raise the right leg and swing it over the left leg. Lift the right leg slightly and dorsi-flex the foot until a pull is felt at the outer thigh. Hold for a count of ten, then release. Repeat with the other leg.
• Supine lying	bend the left knee to the chest, then push the knee across to the right until a pull is felt in the outer thigh. Hold for a count of ten and release. Repeat with the other leg.
• Supine lying	raise the leg to vertical and move it across the body until a pull is felt in the outer thigh. Repeat with the other leg.
• Standing	take the right leg across behind the left as far as possible and place the foot on the ground with the toes turned in. Take the body weight through this leg until a pull is felt in the outer thigh. Hold for a count of ten, then release. Repeat with the other leg.
• Long sitting	bend the right knee and place the foot on the far side of the left leg, level with the knee. Push the bent knee over the left until a pull is felt in the outer thigh. Hold for a count of ten and release. Repeat with the other leg.

Buttock stretching

HIP EXTENSORS: GLUTEUS MAXIMUS

Starting position	Exercise
• Lying	bend the right knee onto the chest, then pull the knee closer, keeping the other leg straight and the back flat against the floor until a pull is felt in the buttock. Hold for a count of ten and release. Repeat with the other leg.
• Inclined prone kneeling	stretch the hands forwards onto the floor, bend the right knee towards the hands, then drop the trunk onto the thigh. Hold for a count of ten and release. Repeat with the other leg. (Caution: not to be done by anyone with knee problems.)
• Standing	bend the right knee to the chest, then pull knee closer, but do not arch the back. Hold for a count of ten and release. Repeat with the other leg.
• Standing	place the right foot on a step, then drop the trunk forward and inside the leg, bending the left knee until a pull is felt in the right buttock. Hold for a count of ten and release. Repeat with the other leg.
• Crook lying	bend the right leg up and place the ankle across the left thigh. Lift the left leg up and back to apply pressure on the right leg until a pull is felt in the right buttock. Hold for a count of ten and release. Repeat with the other leg.

HIP FLEXOR STRETCHING

PSOAS AND ILIACUS, SARTORIUS

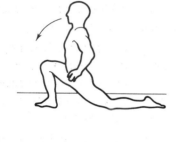

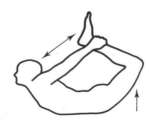

Starting position	Exercise
• Walk standing	bend the forward knee, feeling the pull in the other hip. Repeat with the other leg.
• Supine lying	press one leg firmly against the floor and bend the other leg onto the chest. Pull the bent leg with the hands, feeling the pull in front of the hip on the straight leg. Hold and release. Repeat with the other leg.
• Half kneeling	lean forwards over the bent knee and feel the pull in the other hip. Hold and release. Repeat with the other leg.
• Prone kneeling	lift one leg up behind and place it on a chair with the knee supported. Bend the other knee and let the body move downwards, feeling the stretch on the straight leg. Hold and release. Repeat with the other leg.
• Crook lying	lift the buttocks off the floor, pushing upwards as high as possible. Hold and release.
• Prone lying	bend the knees and grasp the feet with hands, pulling the trunk up. Hold and release. (Caution: this should only be done by the young and flexible.)

LOWER BACK STRETCHING

ERECTOR SPINAE AND QUADRATUS LUMBORUM

Starting position	*Exercise*
• Crook lying	pressing the small of the back into the floor, bring the right knee onto the chest. Clasp the hands around the knee and pull it towards the chest. Hold then relax. Repeat with the other leg.
• Crook lying	pressing the small of the back into the floor, bring both knees onto the chest. Clasp the hands around the thighs and pull them towards the chest. Hold for a count of ten and release.
• Crook lying	as above, but also lift the head and shoulders off the ground. Hold for a count of ten and release.
• Crook lying	keeping the knees together, drop them down to the right, feeling a pull on left side. Hold and release. Then drop the knees to the other side. Hold and release.
• Yard lying	bend the right knee and place the foot outside the left knee. Bring the left hand down and pull the knee to the left, keeping the right arm and shoulder on the floor. Hold and release. Repeat with the other leg.
• Prone kneeling	contract the abdominals and round the back, then lower it to horizontal.
• Crook lying with a firm rolled towel under the sacrum	press the lower back against the floor. Hold and release.
• Sitting with feet on floor	lean the body forward, taking the trunk down to the thighs. Hang the arms at the sides.

ARM STRETCHING

BICEPS, TRICEPS, LATISSIMUS DORSI

Starting position	Exercise
	Biceps stretch
• Stride standing	clasp the hands behind the back. Keeping the elbows straight, raise the arms upwards. Hold for a count of ten and release.
• Stride standing	lift a bar above the head and stretch the arms backwards. Keep the elbows straight.
	Triceps stretch
• Stride standing	lift the right arm upwards and bend the elbow so that the hand lies behind the head. Use the other hand behind the head to push the upper arm down further. Repeat with the other arm.
• Stride standing	clasp the hands above the head, and pull the arms backwards as far as possible behind the head. Hold for a count of ten and release.
	Latissimus dorsi stretch
Stride standing	Lift one arm upwards and bend the elbow so that the hand lies behind the head. Use the other hand to pull the arm towards the body and bend the trunk to the same side. Hold and release. Repeat with the other arm.

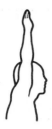

• Stretch stride standing	place the backs of the hands together and stretch towards the ceiling.

FRONT OF THORAX STRETCHING

PECTORALIS MAJOR

Starting position	*Exercise*
• Stride standing	press the shoulders backwards.
• Crook lying, arms at sides	place a tightly-rolled hand towel lengthways between the scapulae. Press the shoulders down into the floor.
• Crook lying, arms out to side, elbows at right angles, palms facing upwards	the same action as above.
• Yard crook lying	the same action as above.
• Prone kneeling	stretch the arms forwards and outwards until the elbows are straight. Extend the wrists and drop the chest forwards, pulling the shoulders backwards.
• Lying with a pillow between the shoulders	raise the arms above the head and press them into the floor.

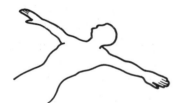

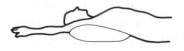

- Stride standing or high sitting

place one bent arm behind the head with the elbow pointing upwards, the other behind the back with the elbow pointing downwards. Clasp the hands if possible, or link them with a towel or strap. Pull downwards, bringing the upper arm back and nearer the head. Repeat with the other arm.

- Stride standing or high sitting

use a bar that is shoulder-width long or just over. Hold the bar at the ends, lift it upwards above the head and then lower it downwards behind the head.

- Long sitting with back to a chair or wall bars

place the arms behind and grasp the sides of the chair. Keep the elbows straight and thrust the chest upwards and forwards, keeping the chin in. Hold then release.

- Standing with back to wall bars

place the arms behind and grasp the wall bar just below shoulder height. Drop the body forward and pull back between the scapulae. Keep the chin in. Hold and release.

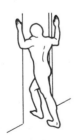

- Walk standing in an open doorway

with the elbows and shoulders at right angles, place one hand on the wall on either side of the doorway. Lean forward into the doorway.

T A S K S

Select exercises from the previous list, and add any of your own:

- Devise exercise schemes for strengthening the following muscles – gastrocnemius; quadriceps; hamstrings; gluteus maximus; abductors; adductors; abdominals; the middle fibres of the trapezius; rhomboids.

- Devise exercise schemes for stretching the following muscles – gastrocnemius; quadriceps; hamstrings; hip flexors; back extensors; pectorals.

- Teach one of your schemes to a partner or group.

Mobility exercises

Neck mobility

Note: keep the shoulders relaxed throughout.

Starting position	Exercise
• Stride standing or sitting	tuck the chin in and drop the head forwards, then lift the chin and take the head backwards. (Caution: do not hyper-extend.)
• Stride standing or sitting	looking straight ahead, take the head sideways, the ear towards the shoulder, first to the right and then to the left.
• Stride standing or sitting	keeping the chin in, turn the head towards the right shoulder and then the left shoulder.
• Stride standing or sitting	tuck the chin in, drop the head forwards and keep the chin on the chest. Then turn the head to the right and then the left.

Do not circle the head round and round as this can damage the cervical joints and cause pressure on the spinal nerves in this area.

Shoulder mobility

Starting position	Exercise
• Stride standing or sitting	pull the shoulders back and relax. Lift the shoulders up and down.
• Stride standing or sitting	circle the shoulders forward, upwards, backwards and down, then the other way.
• Stride standing	swing the arms forwards and up above the head, then down and backwards.
• Stride standing	swing the arms sideways and up to cross above the head, then down to cross behind the back.

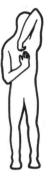

• Stride standing	keep the elbows straight and rotate the arms medially and laterally (turn in and out).
• Stride standing	circle the arms backwards alternately and then together.
• Stride standing	swing the arms backwards alternately and then together.
• Stride standing	raise the arms sideways to clap above the head and then lower them to clap the sides.
• Stride standing	place the right hand behind the neck and the left arm behind the back, trying to touch hands, then change hands.
• Stride standing or sitting	reach forward, keeping the arms at shoulder level, cross the arms and clasp the hands, lift the arms straight above the head and push backwards behind the head.
• Yard stride standing	bend the elbows with the palms facing forward, drop the arms so that the palms face backwards and rotate the arms up and down.

Combinations of the above movements can be used and performed to music. Towels, bars and dumb-bells can be used to add variety and interest.

• Prone kneeling on elbows (not hands)	resting the chin on one hand, take the other arm under the body and stretch it down the outside of opposite leg, then take it out and lift it out to the side. Repeat with the other arm.

TRUNK MOBILITY

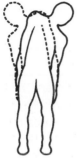

Starting position	Exercise
• Stride standing, hands on thighs	keeping the chin in, curl the trunk forwards while sliding the hands down the thighs.
• Stride standing, hands on buttocks	extend the trunk backwards while sliding the hands down the buttocks.
• Stride standing, hands to sides	bend the trunk to the right and then to the left while sliding the hands down the sides.
• Bend stride standing	twist the trunk to the right and then to the left.
• Reach stride standing	twist the trunk to the right and then to the left.
• Crook lying	pressing the lower back into the floor, bend alternate legs onto the chest.
• Crook lying	bend both legs onto the chest.
• Crook lying	bend both legs onto the chest and lift the head and shoulders towards the knees, clasping the knees with the hands.
• Crook lying	keep the shoulders against the floor. Tip both knees to the right and then to the left. Keep the knees together.
• Supine lying	stretch the right arm down the right side and the left arm down the left side.
• Prone kneeling with back flat	arch the back upwards, pull in the stomach, lower the back and hollow it gently.
• Prone kneeling with back flat	bend the right knee onto the chest, arch the back and kick out behind. Repeat with the left leg. (Caution: perform this exercise carefully, lifting the leg only fifteen degrees above horizontal.)
• Prone kneeling	stretch the opposite arm and leg outwards and upwards. Repeat with the other side.

• Supine lying	lift the right leg to a right angle to the body. Lower the leg towards the floor on the left side of the body, twisting the trunk gently. Repeat with the other leg.
• Prone lying	lift the opposite arm and leg upwards. Repeat on the other side.

HIP MOBILITY

Starting position	Exercise
• Support standing	raise one leg and swing it forwards and backwards. Keep the toes pointing forwards, do not move the trunk and keep the hip forwards. Repeat with the other leg.
• Support standing	raise one leg out sideways and swing it sideways and back across the other leg. Keep the toe pointing forwards and do not move the trunk. Repeat with the other leg.
• Support standing	raise one leg and circle it around. Repeat with the other leg.
• Prone kneeling	bend the knee up to the chest and kick out and up. Repeat with the other leg. (Caution: this should be performed carefully, lifting the leg only fifteen degrees above horizontal.)
• Supine lying	part the legs and bring them together.
• Crook lying	drop the knees outwards and bring them together.
• Supine lying	bend the knees onto the chest and straighten them into the air, keeping them at 90° to the body. Open and cross the legs in a scissor movement. Bend the knees to the chest to lower them.

• Prone lying	bend the knees at a right angle, slightly apart. Swing the feet out sideways and inwards to cross the legs.
• Standing	run on the spot, lifting the knees higher and higher.
• Standing	star jumping – jump feet into stride standing position and back. (Caution: do not abduct too far.)
• Walk standing	bring back foot forwards and take forward foot back by jumping.

KNEE MOBILITY

Starting position	*Exercise*
• High sitting on a chair or the end of a couch	swing the lower legs up and down from bent to straight knee.
• Prone lying on a couch, with feet over the end	bend alternate knees, bringing heel to buttock, and straighten.
• Prone lying on a couch, with feet over the end	bend one knee and cross the other leg over the back of the bent leg. Now push with the back leg to increase the bend in the front leg. This is useful if there is limited range in the knee joint. Repeat with the other leg.
• Supine lying	bend one knee onto the chest. Kick it out straight and lower it. If bending is limited, grasp the knee with hands and pull it into the body. Repeat with the other leg. (Caution: DO NOT perform this exercise with both legs together.)
• Supine lying	bend the knees onto the chest and straighten them into the air. Cycle the legs in the air.
• Support standing	hold onto a wall bar with the hands at shoulder height. Bend the knees and hips down to the squatting position, hold and straighten. (Caution: do not take the buttocks below the knees.)

Use an exercise bike and cycle with the saddle as low as possible.

FOOT MOBILITY

Starting position	Exercise
• Sitting with feet on floor	• push the toes into the floor (do not let them curl); • raise the toes away from the floor; • spread the toes outwards and together; • move the big toes towards each other; • pick up a pencil with the toes.
• Sitting with feet on floor and a towel or strap lengthways under foot	keeping the heel firmly pressed onto towel, use the toes to pull the towel towards the heel.
• Sitting with feet on floor and a towel or strap widthways under foot	keeping the heel on the ground, move the towel to one side and then the other.
• Sitting with hands over top of toes	push down with the hand and lift the toes up against the resistance.
• Sitting with hands under the toes	push up with the hand and push down with the toes against the resistance.
• Sitting with one leg across the other at the knee	turn the foot in and out.
• Sitting with one leg across the other at the knee	pull the foot up and down.
• Sitting with one leg across the other at the knee	circle the foot ten times one way and ten times the opposite way.
• Long sitting	turn the feet inwards and press the inner arches together.

Additional exercises:

- Walk around, moving the weight from the heel to the outer border to the ball of the foot.
- Walk in a straight line, moving the weight from the heel to the outer border to the ball of the foot.
- Walk around on the toes.
- Walk around on the heels.

- Walk normally.
- Skip or jog, changing direction.
- Hop on one leg, then the other.
- Jump forwards, backwards and sideways.
- Jump to stride and back, jump to walk and back, squat jump.

T A S K

Work as a group. Each member of the group must devise and teach five mobility exercises for one named joint. Each person should take a different joint.

CHAPTER 13

Specific exercise programmes

Specific exercise programmes may be required to mobilise joints, to strengthen specific muscles or to correct postural faults.

The objectives must be clearly stated and explained to the client. The client should be encouraged to practise the exercises at home. Consider the starting positions carefully. Younger clients can use standing or modifications of standing, but older clients will be more stable in sitting or lying. Older clients, or those with painful or arthritic joints, should not be placed in the kneeling position.

Careful analysis of the problem areas is necessary so that the appropriate corrective strategy may be worked out. The following are possible exercises for the correction of common problems.

In addition, read the sections on strengthening and stretching, the warm-up and the cool-down in chapter 12. Any appropriate exercises may be selected from those listed, or you may add some of your own. Remember that strength will only improve if the muscle is made to work progressively harder. The intensity of the exercises should increase gradually to peak intensity and decrease gradually. This applies to the warm-up and the main scheme.

The postural correction of lordosis

This is an exaggerated curve of the lumbar spine where the pelvis is tilted forward.

The weak muscles that require strengthening are the abdominals – the rectus abdominus, the internal oblique and the external oblique – and the hip extensors – the hamstrings and the gluteus maximus.

The tight muscles that require stretching are the trunk extensors – the erector spinae and quadratus lumborum – and the hip flexors, particularly the ilio-psoas.

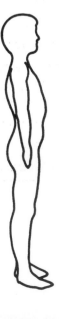

Figure 13.1 *Lordosis*

AIMS OF THE TREATMENT

- To strengthen the abdominals, thus pulling the pelvis upwards and backwards
- To strengthen the hip extensors
- To stretch the erector spinae and quadratus lumborum
- To stretch the hip flexors.

Remember to use crook lying as a starting position for the abdominal strengthening and to keep the small of the back against the floor.

EXERCISES

Read the appropriate suggestions for strengthening and stretching in chapters 11 and 12.

SAMPLE SCHEME

WARM-UP - INCLUDE EXERCISES FOR MOBILISING, PULSE RAISING AND SHORT STRETCH

Starting position	Exercise
• Support standing	leg swinging forward and back.
• Stride standing	hips rotation.
• Stride standing	flex trunk to right and left.
• Stride standing	trunk twist to right and left.
• Stride standing with lax knees	pull pelvis upwards and relax.
• Stride standing	shoulder rolls.
• Stride standing	stepping forwards, back and sideways accompanied by arm movements.
• stride standing	stepping with kick.
• Stride standing	stretch.
• Standing	hold posture correction.

MAIN CORRECTIVE SCHEME

Starting position	Exercise
• Crook lying	tilt pelvis, upwards pressing the lumbar region into the floor, release.
• Crook lying	keeping the chin in, raise the head and shoulders to look at the knees.
• Crook lying	curl up. This is progressed by moving the hand position to head rest and then stretching above the head.
• Bend crook lying	twist the trunk, bringing alternate elbows to the opposite knee.
• Yard crook lying	drop the knees to the right and then to the left.
• Lying	slide the right arm down the right side and the left arm down the left side.
• Prone kneeling	arch the back to stretch the lumbar spine, then return to horizontal.
• Prone kneeling	stretch alternate legs out and lift no more than fifteen degrees above horizontal.

COOL-DOWN

Starting position	Exercise
• Yard lying	bend the right knee and place the foot outside the left knee. Bring the left hand down and pull bent knee across to the left, keeping the right arm and shoulder on the floor. Hold for a count of ten, then release. Repeat on the other side.
• Crook lying	place a firm rolled towel under the sacrum. Press the lower back against the floor, hold for a count of ten, then release.
• Half kneeling	lean forwards over the bent knee and feel a pull in the front of the opposite hip. Hold for a count of ten and release.

• Stride standing	pull in the abdomen and release.
• Stride standing	rotate the pelvis.
• Standing	gentle heel raise then jog with arm swinging.
• Walking	arm upstretch (shoulder press).
• Lying	breathe deeply, pulling in the abdomen with exhalation.

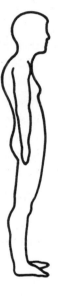

Figure 13.2 *Kyphosis*

The postural correction of kyphosis

This is an exaggerated curve of the thoracic region. The shoulders are usually rounded, the neck is shortened and held in extension and the chin pokes forward.

The weak muscles that require strengthening are the middle fibres of the trapezius, the rhomboids and the erector spinae.

The tight muscles that require stretching are the pectoralis major and the neck extensors.

AIMS OF THE TREATMENT

- To strengthen the shoulder retractors, namely the middle fibres of the trapezius and the rhomboids, thus drawing the shoulders backwards
- To strengthen the erector spinae to maintain the erect posture
- To stretch the pectoralis major.

Remember that many of these exercises are also used to correct round shoulders. Always keep the chin in and maintain a long neck when performing these exercises.

EXERCISES

Read the appropriate suggestions for strengthening and stretching in chapters 11 and 12.

SAMPLE SCHEME

WARM-UP – MOBILISERS, PULSE
RAISERS, STRETCH. MAIN
CORRECTIVE SCHEME

Starting position	Exercise
• Standing	hold posture correction.
• Stride standing	gently drop the head forward, pulling the chin in. Press the head back, making a long neck, and raise.
• Lax stoop sitting	raise the trunk gradually from the base of the spine, vertebra by vertebra.
• Lax stoop sitting	as above, against resistance from the therapist.
• Stride standing	circle the shoulders backwards.
• Stride standing	circle the arms backwards.
• Stride standing	pull the shoulders backwards.
• Across bend stride standing	pull the shoulders back and release. Then pull the elbows back and release. Then press the arms back and release.
• Lax stoop stride standing	slowly return to standing from the base of the spine, vertebra by vertebra.
• Stoop standing	clasp the hands behind the back, pull the arms and shoulders up and back, hold for a count of ten and release.
• Prone lying	keeping the chin in, pull the shoulders back and raise the head and shoulders.
• Prone lying, hands clasped behind the back	pull on the hands and pull the shoulders off the floor.
• Prone lying, hands clasped behind back	keeping the chin in, pull the shoulders back, lifting the head and shoulders off the floor.

• Wing prone lying	keeping the chin in, lift the head and shoulders off the floor, pulling the shoulders back.
• Wing prone lying	as above, but against the resistance of the therapist.
• Prone lying	with the arms abducted, elbows bent and palms to the floor, lift the arms and head and shoulders.
• Yard prone lying	as above.

COOL-DOWN

Starting position	*Exercise*
• Crook lying	place a tightly rolled towel lengthways along the spine between the scapulae, press the shoulders back towards the floor, hold for a count of ten and release.
• Crook lying, arms out to side, elbows at right angles, palms facing forward	as above.
• Yard crook lying	as above.
• Sitting	place one hand behind the neck and the other behind the back, and try to clasp hands or link with a strap. Pull downwards, bringing the upper arm nearer the head, hold for a count of ten and release.
• Sitting	use a bar that is shoulder-width long. Hold the bar at the ends, lift it upwards above the head and then lower it down behind the head. Hold for a count of ten and lift up.
• Prone kneeling	raise alternate arms sideways and upwards.
• Jogging	gentle jogging, circling arms backwards.
• Walking	walking around swinging arms.
• Lying	deep breathing.

Kyphosis–lordosis is a combination of the previous two conditions. Select exercises from the two schemes for this condition.

The postural correction of round shoulders

In this condition the shoulders are protracted (drawn forward), the head is extended and the chin pokes forward.

This postural defect may be present without any kyphosis of the spine. However, if the spine is kyphotic the shoulders will also be rounded.

The weak muscles that require strengthening are the middle fibres of the trapezius and the rhomboids.

The tight muscles that require stretching are the pectorals and the neck extensors.

AIMS OF THE TREATMENT

- To strengthen the shoulder retractors and draw the shoulders backwards
- To stretch the pectoralis major and the neck extensors.

For suitable exercises, refer to the scheme for kyphosis. The same exercises can be used for both conditions.

You may wish to modify this slightly by selecting others from chapters 11 and 12 or by adding your own.

The postural correction of scoliosis

This is a lateral curvature of the spine, which may be a long C curve or an S curve. The condition may cause scapular deviation and slight unevenness in the levels of the shoulders and pelvic girdle, caused by muscle imbalance on the right and left sides of the spine. The spine must be carefully examined. To make observation easier, run a finger downwards along the spinous processes with slight pressure. The red line will show the extent and direction of the curve. If the condition is postural, the curve will right itself in forward flexion; ask the client to bend over so that you can see if this is so. If the condition does not correct with flexion it is a structural problem and should be referred to a doctor.

The muscles that will require strengthening will be those on the outside of the curve. The muscles that will require stretching will be those on the inside of the curve.

General back-strengthening exercises are usually effective in correcting this condition. It is frequently found in adolescence, when pupils carry heavy school bags over the same shoulder or in the same hand each day. Suggest that the bag is carried in one hand to school and in the other on the way home.

AIMS OF THE TREATMENT

To restore balance to muscles of the back, thus reducing the deformity.

EXERCISES

WARM-UP

Read suggestions for strengthening erector spinae.

Warm-up exercises – mobilisers, pulse raisers and short stretch.

MAIN CORRECTIVE SCHEME

Starting position	Exercise
• Stride standing	reach up into the air with the hand on the concave side of the curve, where the muscles are tight, and reach towards the floor with the other hand. Stretch, hold, relax, repeat.
• Stride standing	side flex the trunk towards the convex side, where the muscles are stretched. Slide the hand down the side and return.
• Prone lying	stretch the arm up along the floor on the concave side and slide the arm down the side of convexity. Hold, release and repeat.
• Prone lying	stretch the arm above the head on the concave side and the opposite leg along the floor.
• Prone lying	raise the opposite arm and leg as above.
• Crook lying, arms abducted and elbows at right angles, palms to floor	rotate the arms to palms up and push back into the floor.
• Prone lying, arms abducted and elbows at right angles, palms to floor	raise arms backwards.

• Prone lying, arms to side	keeping the chin in, lift the head and shoulders.
• Prone lying, clasping hands	keeping the chin in, lift the head and shoulders and pull down the arms.
• Prone lying, arms abducted, elbows at right angles, palms to floor	raise the arms, head and shoulders. (Do not extend the head; keep it in line with the body.)
• Yard prone lying	as above.
• Stretch prone lying	as above.

COOL-DOWN

Select exercises from the previous schemes. Include plenty of shoulder and trunk movements.

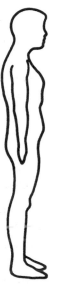

Figure 13.3 *Flat back*

The postural correction of flat back

This is a condition where there is little or no lumbar curve, the back is flat in this region and the pelvis is tilted backwards. It is usually accompanied by kyphosis of the thoracic spine.

The muscles that require strengthening are the back extensors, namely the erector spinae. (Sometimes the abdominals and gluteus maximus are weak.) The muscles that require stretching are the hamstrings.

AIMS OF THE TREATMENT

- To try to develop a normal lumbar curve by strengthening the erector spinae and gluteus maximus
- To maintain a correct pelvic tilt by ensuring the strength of the abdominals and stretch of the hamstrings.

EXERCISES

WARM-UP – MOBILISERS, PULSE RAISERS AND STRETCH

Select any warm-up exercises from the previous schemes.

MAIN CORRECTIVE SCHEME

Starting position	Exercise
• Sitting	lean forward, taking the pressure from the buttocks onto the thigh, then extend the back to create a lumbar lordosis. Hold for a count of ten and release.
• Prone lying	raise alternate legs.
• Prone lying	raise both legs (allowed for this condition).
• Prone kneeling	arch and hollow the back.
• Prone kneeling	lift alternate legs up and backwards, stretch, hold and return to the floor.
• Lying with rolled towel under lumbar spine	flex one knee, then extend the leg up towards the ceiling. Keep the opposite leg pressed hard down on the floor. Repeat with the other leg.
• Long sitting	rotate the pelvis forwards, then lean slightly backwards. Hold and release.
• Supine lying, legs up against a wall, with a towel under lumbar spine	pull alternate legs away from the wall, keeping the knee straight and the pelvis on the floor. Hold and release.

COOL-DOWN

Any exercises as previous schemes.

The correction of flabby upper arms

This is due to poor muscle tone in the triceps, which is the extensor muscle of the elbow. Fatty deposits in this area also contribute to the problem.

The muscle that requires strengthening is the triceps. If the client is overweight, he or she will need aerobic work to reduce the percentage of body fat.

AIMS OF THE TREATMENT

- To increase the strength of the triceps muscle
- To reduce body fat if necessary.

Remember that the triceps extends the elbow joint; therefore, elbow extension must be the movement that is included in all exercises for improving this condition. Movement downwards is assisted by gravitational pull and uses the biceps, working eccentrically, to control the movement, so that the triceps is not working. Movements using the triceps must therefore be horizontal or upwards.

EXERCISES

WARM-UP – MOBILISERS, PULSE RAISERS AND STRETCH

If the client needs to lose weight, include an aerobic section here for twenty minutes.

MAIN CORRECTIVE SCHEME

Starting position	Exercise
• Across bend sitting or stride standing	stretch alternate arms out sideways and back; stretch both arms out sideways and back.
• Bend stride standing	punch forward; punch a pillow or punch bag.
• Stride standing	place the hands against the therapist's hands, with elbows bent. Push alternate arms straight against the therapist's resistance.
• Bend stride standing or sitting	stretch the arm vertically upwards. Repeat with progressive weights.

- Stride standing, arms bent, hands against a wall, leaning forwards   push away from the wall.

- Prone kneeling   bend and straighten the elbows.

- Prone lying   place the hands under the shoulders and push up.

- Prone lying   press-ups.

- Lean sitting holding weights   holding the weight in the hand at shoulder level, extend the arm backwards and upwards.

- Crook lying   holding the weight in the hands at shoulder level, push the weights vertically upward and then lower. The weights can be increased for progression.

COOL-DOWN

Starting position	Exercise
• Walking	walking around the room, bending and stretching the elbows.
• Stepping forward and back	punch the arms forward or chest press.
• Standing	alternate heel raising combined with shoulder shrugging.
• Sitting	circle the shoulders.
• Bend sitting	reach alternate arms forwards and sideways.
• Sitting	shake the arms.
• Lying	deep breathing.

The correction of winged scapula

This is a condition where the medial border and inferior angle of the scapula move back away from the chest wall. It is due to weakness of the serratus anterior and the lower fibres of the trapezius.

Muscles that require strengthening are the serratus anterior and the lower fibres of the trapezius.

AIMS OF THE TREATMENT

- To strengthen those muscles which hold the scapula against the chest wall.

Remember that the serratus anterior is used powerfully in all punching movements. It helps the trapezius to swing the scapula laterally during arm abduction and arm swinging, and it works powerfully to hold the scapula in position when the weight of the body is taken on the hands, as in prone kneeling, push-ups and press-ups.

The exercises for strengthening this muscle are the same as those for strengthening the triceps (pages 218–219).

The correction of flabby buttocks

These are caused by poor muscle tone in the hip extensors, primarily the gluteus maximus. The hip abductors also contribute to the problem, namely the gluteus medius, gluteus minimus and tensor fascia lata.

The muscles that require strengthening are the hip extensors, i.e. the gluteus maximus, the hamstrings and the hip abductors.

The muscles that require stretching are the hip flexors, primarily the ilio-psoas.

AIMS OF THE TREATMENT

- To increase the strength of the hip extensors and abductors
- To stretch the hip flexors.

Remember that the hip extensors will extend the fully flexed hip backwards until the leg is in line with the body and for a further fifteen degrees. At this point further movement is prevented by the structure and ligaments of the hip joint and by the tension in the flexors. The hip extensors will also pull the forward-flexed trunk upwards, working with origin and insertion reversed.

EXERCISES

WARM-UP – MOBILISERS, PULSE
RAISERS, STRETCH. MAIN
CORRECTIVE SCHEME

Starting position	Exercise
• High sitting	tighten the buttocks.
• High sitting	press the thighs downwards into the seat and rotate them outwards.
• Forward stoop sitting	raise the trunk upwards against the resistance of the therapist.
• Stoop stride standing, hands on legs	raise the trunk to standing.
• Crook lying	tighten the buttocks and raise the pelvis.
• Prone kneeling	stretch alternate legs out behind. Attach ankle weights for progression. (Caution: do not arch the back or lift the leg more than fifteen degrees above horizontal.)
• Side lying	swing the legs forward and back.
• Side lying	push back against resistance from the therapist or springs.
• Side lying	raise and lower the upper leg, using weights for progression.
• Prone lying	bending the knee, raise alternate legs off the floor.
• Prone lying	raise alternate legs off the floor (Caution: extend the leg fifteen degrees only and keep the hips on the floor.) Use weights for progression.
• Prone lying on a couch with one leg over the edge	lift this leg backwards and upwards fifteen degrees from horizontal. Use weights for progression. Repeat with the other leg.

COOL-DOWN

- Skipping
- Marching with arm swinging

- Stride standing, lower and raise the trunk. (Caution: do not bend the knees beyond a right angle)
- Jog around the room
- Step swing forward, back, side with elbow flexion and extension
- Buttock clenching while sitting
- In supine lying, bend one knee onto the chest, hug it with the hands and push the straight leg into the ground. Repeat with the other leg
- Deep breathing while lying

T A S K S

Work with a partner. Practise a role play with one of you as the client and the other as the therapist.

- Select one of the postural problems – the 'client' mimics this standing posture.
- Identify the weak muscles for strengthening and the tight muscles for stretching.

- Construct a scheme of exercises to correct the problem.
- Teach the exercises to the client.

CHAPTER 14

Exercise classes

Exercise classes provide many different forms of exercise, for example general keep fit, aerobic, dance, step, weight loss, relaxation, etc. Although they differ in the type of exercise offered, certain basic principles apply to all.

It is desirable, though not always possible, to organise classes so that there is parity within the groups, for example similar fitness levels, similar age groups and similar desired outcomes. It is very important to recognise and allow for individual differences within a group: different intellectual levels, fitness levels, body shapes, health, previous experience, lifestyles, age and motivation.

Each class member must be instructed to work at his or her own pace, and heart rate must be used to monitor intensity. No-one should exceed their maximum heart rate (see page 96). Remember: beginners must work at 60 per cent of the maximum heart rate and increase to 80 per cent as fitness develops. All members must practice taking the radial pulse for fifteen seconds and multiplying by four. They must continue to monitor the pulse at intervals throughout the class. Members must stop exercising if the maximum heart rate is exceeded or if there are any signs of stress.

Learning new skills

The theories of learning apply to both individual and class teaching. Members attend in order to acquire new skills, which will aid the achievement of set goals or objectives. These goals will vary from person to person. In order to help the members of a class to achieve these goals, the teacher must organise the lessons so that optimum learning and performance can take place.

The teaching of a skill requires demonstration (by the teacher) followed by practice by the members, but before this can occur it is essential to prepare adequately the environment where the learning is to take place.

As previously outlined, the environment must be warm, well ventilated, free from distractions and external noise and safe. The floor must be firm, smooth and, preferably, sprung. All equipment must be checked and organised before the commencement of the class so that the sequence of the lesson is not broken, as interruption of any kind interferes with the learning process. Members must be acknowledged and greeted in a friendly and reassuring way. This ensures that members feel physically and psychologically 'safe'.

Learning a new exercise is a very complex process. It is useful to consider the nature of a skill and how it may be defined.

- Curzon (1976) defines a skill as 'a series of learned acts requiring simultaneous or sequential co-ordination'.
- The UK Department of Employment (Curzon, 1976) defines a skill as 'an organised and co-ordinated pattern of mental and physical activity'.

The essential features of a skilled performance are:

- accuracy of timing;
- anticipation of movement;
- economy of effort;
- grace and precision of movement;
- the overall flow of the movement.

To enable members of the class to attain this level, the teacher must analyse each skill and break it down into a sequence of separate movements, which are then joined together to make the whole performance. The acquisition of a skill requires the use of both receptor and effector processes, in other words effective co-ordination of mind and muscle. There are many theories on the learning of motor skills.

Other theories suggest that the learner must pass through three overlapping phases:

- The *cognitive phase* – this involves knowledge of the skill. The learner analyses the task and tries to understand what is to be done. He or she knows when errors are made but is unsure how to correct them. At this stage cues and correction must be given frequently and common errors pointed out.
- The *associative phase* – as a result of practice, errors are gradually eliminated. Correct patterns are established and, although errors are still made, they are corrected with minimal prompting.

- The *autonomous phase* – skills are performed automatically and require little thought. Errors have been eliminated, speed and accuracy increased and the effects of stress reduced.

FEEDBACK

It is the instructor's role to guide members of the class through these stages and to provide continuous feedback throughout. They must be informed of their current progress and told how to improve it. Millar distinguishes between two forms of feedback:

- *Action feedback*, which provides knowledge of current progress. Actions are corrected as they are performed. The instructor must therefore provide spoken cues during the performance of the exercise, such as 'eyes front', 'hold the head up', 'shoulders down', 'knees higher', 'do not stretch too far', 'do not lift too high', 'curl back slowly from below', etc.

- *Learning feedback*, which provides information that enables the student to improve next time. This might include cues such as 'that was a good attempt, but some people did not keep the back straight', 'well done, but keep those tummies in', 'well done, but watch that you roll the pelvis backwards before you come up' or 'I obviously didn't explain that exercise clearly', followed by further explanation and demonstration. In this way, members can correct their performance and will move quickly into the autonomous phase.

Feedback must therefore be given as each exercise or part of an exercise is being performed, and also at the end. This enables the learner to discriminate between correct and incorrect patterns at an early stage and thus avoids incorrect patterns being reinforced.

Many corrective statements and cues will be required for new members of a class or when members are learning a new exercise, but as the skill is mastered fewer cues are needed. Positive value statements such as 'good', 'that's better', 'well done' or 'great' will encourage members and increase motivation. It is important always to encourage and never to put anyone down, nor draw attention to poor performance or embarrass the learner. If only one or two members are not performing correctly, give a general corrective statement, or catch their eye and say 'watch me', or explain the correction quietly and privately at the end of the class.

Feedback is essential as it provides knowledge of correct or incorrect performance, reinforces the correct response and increases motivation.

Motivation

Motivation may be defined as the drive within an individual to take an appropriate course of action in order to satisfy a need.

Motivation heightens performance. The good instructor, teacher or coach is able to stimulate the student's own motivation. The instructor can ensure that the class is well organised and administered and that the teaching style is enthusiastic, positive, concerned, caring, knowledgeable and safe. A high level of expertise must be demonstrated at all times, both in theoretical knowledge and in practical demonstration.

Motivation is greatly enhanced by encouraging and promoting feelings of satisfaction, achievement, recognition, responsibility, advancement, personal growth and success.

However, poor, unpleasant surroundings, lack of organisation and safety, feelings of dissatisfaction, failure and embarrassment, lack of interest and unrealistic goals that are not achievable are all demotivators and must be avoided.

SETTING OBJECTIVES OR GOALS

This is a very important part of planning for group or individual exercises. The members' aspirations and the possibilities of realising them must be fully discussed. When members are involved in setting the objectives they know where they are going and can better help themselves to get there, so motivation is increased. The objective may be to:

- increase cardio-respiratory fitness;
- improve muscle strength;
- improve flexibility;
- reduce fatty deposits;
- improve body shape;
- improve posture;
- correct figure faults;
- improve speed and skill.

Objectives must be realistic and they must be achievable within a limited time scale. A rounded five foot tall endomorph will never be tall and slender – that goal would be unrealistic – but to lose fat and improve body shape would be achievable and realistic. The setting of long-term goals and short-term goals, which are continually monitored through regular assessment, will increase motivation. Once the objectives have been agreed, planning the strategy can begin. Lesson plans for each session should be prepared: these are necessary as a record of work and show progression.

Each lesson plan should include:

- the objectives;
- the sequence of activities;
- the time allowed for each part of the sequence;
- the music, if used;
- the equipment necessary;
- any comments or notes.

An example can be found in Table 14.1.

Objective:
- To correct lordosis and improve muscle balance
- To reduce weight.

Table 14.1 *Sample lesson plan*

Activity	Time	Equipment	Music	Comments
Discussion of previous week's class including any problems, and outline today's exercises	10 minutes	—	—	explain that these objectives require different exercises: • to reduce weight – aerobics; • to correct lordosis – strengthening abdominals and stretching back extensors
Warm-up: alternate heel raising, walking on the spot and around the room, marching with knees high, pelvic tilt, circle pelvis, twist trunk, shoulder circling, arm circling, chest press	10 minutes	—	any suitable music for age group or time of year	begin slowly and increase pace. Work on large muscle groups. Include exercises for mobilising and pulse raising
Stretch: erector spinae, hip flexors (select from chapter 12)	5 minutes	rolled towel	—	slow gentle static stretch, hold for a count of ten, repeat
Aerobic section	15 minutes	step	theme music, faster tempo	work to target heart rate. Take pulse every five minutes, stop if above target, work harder if too low (see chapter 8)

| Strengthening exercises | 10 minutes | medicine ball, sand bag | — | use crook lying curl-ups for the abdominal muscles and leg extension for the gluteus maximus and hamstrings. Caution: do not extend the lower back, keep the hips on the floor |
| Cool-down: select from chapter 12. Stretch | 10 minutes | — | any music with a slow tempo | keep moving – do not stand still |

The organisation of a class

- Prepare the room before the members arrive.
- Ensure that the lighting and ventilation are adequate.
- Check that the floor is firm, clean and smooth.
- Locate the first-aid box and note all the exits.
- Check that the area is clear of equipment or apparatus or anything that may be a safety hazard.
- Select all required equipment or apparatus.
- Check that the equipment and apparatus is in sound working order.
- Arrange all the equipment neatly at one end of the room well away from the working area.
- Select the music tapes or records and stack them in order of use.
- Check that the music centre or player is working.
- Provide a large clock with a second hand to be used when monitoring maximum heart rate.
- Shower and change into appropriate clothes. Remember that you set the standard for the class. Wear clean, unrestricting, absorbent, smart clothing and suitable footwear (see chapter 10).
- Tie the hair back and remove jewellery.

When the members arrive:

- Greet the members warmly, using their names where possible; at the very least, make eye contact or wave to show each member that they are recognised.
- Make a point of greeting and speaking to new members.

- Carry out a consultation or assessment of each new member and ensure that he or she has read the instructions (see chapter 10) and signed the consent form.
- Check that members are wearing suitable unrestricting clothing and suitable footwear.
- Check that hair is tied back and jewellery is removed.
- Begin the class on time.

During the class:

- Step confidently in front of the class, speak clearly and make sure that those at the back can hear. Use the voice to good effect: change the tone to govern speed, rhythm, intensity and effort.
- Remember that you are the role model for the class. Therefore, develop a warm, friendly, enthusiastic, positive approach. Good posture and an alert and efficient manner will set the tone of the class. Do not fidget or develop irritating mannerisms such as tossing the hair or rubbing the leg.
- When demonstrating an exercise, ensure that your performance is as accurate and perfect as possible. Poor demonstration means poor performance and ineffective exercise, which may also impose stresses on the body, causing strain and injury.
- Become an educator. Explain the reasons for and the effects of each exercise. Explain the health benefits of exercise (see chapter 1).
- Following the demonstration, give clear, simple commands and corrective cues, particularly in the early stages.
- Break complicated exercises down into manageable 'chunks'. Teach one part at a time until each is well executed and then perform them together as a whole.
- Give encouragement to enhance motivation, i.e. 'well done', 'that's good', 'much better', 'that's great', 'a great effort', etc.
- Take time to explain and teach new exercises.
- Stress that each individual must work at his or her own pace. He or she must not exceed the maximum heart rate. New members should work at 60 per cent of MHR working up to 80–85 per cent (see chapter 8).
- Stop exercising if there are signs of stress such as profuse sweating, breathlessness, tightness in the chest, pain in the chest or arms, pain in the back or any joints, faintness or dizziness, headache, nausea or a heart rate above the maximum.
- Members must not be made to feel that they are in competition with others, nor under pressure to keep up with the instructor. If possible, organise classes into easy, intermediate and

advanced to accommodate fitness levels, or organise them into age groups, in order to maintain some parity within the groups. Allow time for discussion before the session commences. This may cover any problems experienced during or after the previous class, any minor injuries or joint problems experienced or any interesting new information for discussion. Explain the importance of maintaining good posture and give advice on protecting the back, neck and knees. (For example, instruct members to go from standing to lying by going down on the hands and knees, rolling onto their side and then onto the back, with the reverse procedure for standing up again.)

- Explain the importance of breathing normally and not holding the breath. Instruct members to breathe in before an effort or on release and to breathe out on the effort.

- Give reasons for the importance of the warm-up (see chapter 12). Emphasise that even if members turn up late they must not join the class until they have completed the ten-minute warm-up. They must do this at the edge or back of the class and then join in the other exercises. Explain the importance of stretching and the associated hazards (see chapter 8).

- Explain the importance of the cool-down in allowing the body to return slowly to the balanced state. Explain why cool-down exercises should be performed while lying down or while continuously moving around.

Aerobic class

The American College of Sports Medicine defines aerobic activity as follows:

> 'Aerobic activity is that requiring continuous, rhythmic use of large muscle groups at 60–90 per cent of the maximum heart rate and 50–85 per cent of maximum oxygen uptake for 20–60 minutes at least three times per week.'

The main effects of aerobic exercises are:

- an increase in cardio-respiratory fitness;
- a reduction of fatty deposits, with resultant weight loss;
- an increase in muscular endurance;
- the maintenance of bone mass.

Types of aerobic class

There are various activities designed to keep the body in continuous rhythmic motion and the list is continually growing.

We now have high, moderate and low impact aerobics, step, dance and water aerobics.

High-impact aerobics, where both feet leave the ground, are no longer recommended as they place members at risk of injury due to continuous jarring. Low impact, where one foot always stays in contact with the ground and the knees are slightly bent, are safer. Moderate impact will include some high impact, but consists mainly of low-impact work. It is more desirable to concentrate on duration and intensity than on impact.

Duration is increased by performing more repetitions. Intensity is increased by using longer and higher steps: from jogging to marching to high stepping. The arm position can change from waist level or at the sides to shoulder level and above the head. Light ankle and wrist weights can be used. Fitter members can exaggerate their movements, taking bigger steps and travelling more.

Energy expenditure will depend on the intensity and duration of the exercises. The higher, faster and longer the movements, the greater will be the energy expenditure.

As with all classes, it is important to begin gradually. This allows the body to adapt to increased demand. Exercises should begin with low-intensity work, build up to peak intensity and decrease gradually.

- The heart must adapt to maintain adequate blood supply to the working muscles.
- Blood flow will be diverted from the organs to the muscles.
- The respiratory rate must increase gradually to ensure adequate ventilation. A too-rapid increase in breathing will result in hyper-ventilation and side cramps.

Plan the class as outlined on pages 227–229. Always include a warm-up, stretching, main core exercises and a cool-down. Relaxation and breathing exercises may also be included if appropriate.

SELECTING MUSIC

Selecting music is an important part of the planning. The music will set the 'mood' of the class, it provides timing for the exercises and it keeps the class working together. It helps to provide interest, fun and enjoyment, and also increases motivation. When selecting music, consider the age range and lifestyle of the clients where possible; for example, younger clients will enjoy contemporary pop music, while older clients may prefer 1960s music, big bands, folk, country and western, gospel or square dance music. Consider also the time of year, for example Christmas music or summer songs. If the class is mixed, use a variety of music, with something to suit everyone. Ask class members if they have favourite records or tapes that they would like to use.

PLANNING EXERCISES TO MUSIC

The choreography, that is the planning of the movements and sequences of music, must be done well in advance. This is difficult at first, but becomes easier with practice. Watch exercise videos, noting how the steps match the beat of the music. Watch modern dance and ballet, observing how foot, trunk and arm movements fit the music.

List all the foot and leg movements that you may wish to include in the class. Then list all the arm movements that may be performed on their own or to accompany the leg movements. For examples, see Table 14.2.

Table 14.2 *Sample lesson plan*

Leg movement	Arm movement
Heel raise	Hands on waist (wing)
Jog	Hands on shoulders (bend)
March	Arms out to side or front
High knee march	Arms on head
Walk	Arms reach up (shoulder press)
Steps forward, back, to side	Alternate arms reach up
Step touches	Alternate arms reach sideways or forwards (chest press)
Step and kick	Swinging forward and back
Step and knee lift	Sideways clap
Step, knee lift and kick	Shoulder shrugging
Plié (caution)	Shoulder circling
Grapevine (cross one leg in front of or behind the other	Air punching forwards and upwards
Hopscotch	Across body swing
Rabbit hops	

In the same way list floor and stretch exercises.

Select music to suit the class. Listen carefully to each piece of music and note:

- the rhythm – this is the regular pattern of sound which will dictate the style of the exercise routine;
- the beat – these are the pulsations of music. The beat is very important as a step or movement will accompany each beat;
- the timing or number of beats in each bar. Music with two or four beats in the bar is best for class work. Waltz time (three beats in a bar) can be used for stretching;
- the tempo – the rate at which the music is played. The American book *Aerobics Dance-Exercise* suggests that slow tempos of 100–120 beats per minute are suitable for warm-up and cool-down, and under 100 beats per minute for stretch and floor exercises, while faster tempos of 130–160 should be used for aerobics and dance.

Having listened to the music, select from the list of exercises suitable movements and patterns to fit the music. Practise these thoroughly yourself and record each movement and series of movements. Movements or patterns are usually repeated four to six times. Plan movements for the warm-up, stretch, main core – building up the intensity and then easing down again – and cool-down. Note cues for good posture, breathing and accurate movements.

Task 1

Work with a partner.

- Prepare a first lesson plan for a 30-year-old client who wants to lose weight and improve the strength of the abdominals.

- Explain the reasons for your choice of exercises to the client.

Task 2

Work with a partner.

- Prepare a working area for an aerobics class.
- Instruct a client on how to lie down on the floor and come up again.

- Teach a client correct breathing, using the diaphragm and lower ribs.

TASK 3

- Plan an aerobics lesson for a group of 30–45-year-olds who are moderately fit.

- Discuss the reasoning behind your selection of exercises.

TASK 4

Work in a group.

- Teach any six exercises to the group without music.

TASK 5

Work in a group.

- Select a piece of suitable music and plan a sequence of movements to fit the music which may be used in an aerobics class.
- Teach these exercises to a small group.

Remember to:

- listen to the music first;

- demonstrate the movement correctly;
- break the movement down into parts;
- teach each part thoroughly, with and without music;
- link all the parts together;
- practise the entire sequence.

CHAPTER 15

Sports injuries

First-aid treatment

The field of sports medicine is vast and highly specialised, and is not within the scope of this book. No-one should attempt to diagnose or treat any injury without medical training. For full recovery accurate diagnosis is crucial, followed by careful rehabilitation. The rate of recovery and return to full function will depend on these factors. Inappropriate treatment can cause further damage and permanently impair function. However, knowing what action to take immediately, before medical attention is available, can reduce the extent of tissue damage. Everyone connected with sport should be familiar with the following principles.

> Immediate action – think 'RICED' and apply appropriate treatments from this list:

- **R** for rest and immobilisation to prevent further damage
- **I** for ice, applied immediately for vasoconstriction
- **C** for compression to the area to reduce swelling
- **E** for elevation, using gravity to assist drainage of exudate from the area
- **D** for diagnosis by a doctor – on site, in a surgery or in hospital

REST AND SUPPORT

Further damage to an injured area can be prevented by resting and immobilising the part. The casualty should only be moved if absolutely necessary: to facilitate breathing, to remove him or her from the field of play or to prevent further injury.

The injured part should be rested and supported correctly, using splints, stocking or crêpe bandages. The strapping, must not be too tight, as it will restrict the circulation and cause further damage. If the swelling increases under the strapping, more pressure will be applied to the blood vessels, causing further restriction. Check the colour of the skin and nails beyond the strapping: white or grey skin and blue nails indicate that the strapping is too tight. Use stretch strapping, which can give as the swelling increases. The arms and legs can be supported using rigid or inflatable splints, tubular or stocking bandages pulled over the area, using two layers for firmer support, or crêpe bandages – these give firmer support if a layer of cotton wool is wrapped around the area before applying the bandage. If a leg fracture is suspected, the good leg can be used as a splint by tying the two legs together, or long strips of wood can be used and bound to the leg.

If the arm is seriously injured, a sling is used for support. A triangular sling is placed around the lower arm, supporting the elbow. The outside corner is taken over the opposite shoulder and the inside corner over the shoulder on the injured side, and the two ends are tied at the back of the neck. If the injury is below the elbow, the forearm should be supported with the hand higher than the elbow, to assist drainage.

CRUTCH WALKING

The casualty should not put weight on an injured leg. Elbow or axillary crutches should be used, or support can be given by a person on either side with the casualty hopping on the good leg.

Measure the crutches carefully. There should be a space the width of three fingers between the top of the crutch and the axilla (armpit), otherwise pressure will damage the nerves in the region. The hand rest should be level with the crease of the wrist or the styloid process.

Two-point walking should be used: both crutches are moved forward together, then the casualty pushes down on the hand rest and straightens the elbows and hops to the crutches. Do not hop through the crutches as this can result in a loss of balance and falling backwards. Do not place the crutches too far forward, as they will slip. Going upstairs, move the foot first, then the crutches; coming downstairs, move the crutches first then the foot.

Elbow crutches are used in a similar way, but do not give as much support.

ICE THERAPY OR CRYOTHERAPY

Ice should be placed over the injured area as soon as possible. Cold will reduce internal bleeding and swelling, as the blood vessels constrict, reducing fluid and bruising.

Care must be taken when applying ice to the area, as there is a risk of producing ice burns if the ice comes into contact with the skin for a prolonged period. The area should be covered with oil, or a tea towel should be used between the skin and the ice.

There arc various ways of applying ice. These include stroking the oiled skin with an ice cube, keeping the ice moving over the area slowly. Alternatively, ice cubes can be shattered and placed in a towel, which is then wrapped around the injury over a tea towel. Freezer packs, or even frozen food such as a packet of peas, can be used. These are placed over a tea towel covering the area and held in place by another towel. These packs are very useful, as they can be refrozen and reused. Ankle and wrist injuries can be immersed in iced water in a bucket or bowl. The part is held in the water for as long as is tolerable, then removed for a few minutes and re-immersed.

Ice should be applied for at least ten to fifteen minutes, unless the skin is sensitive and the area feels uncomfortable. Pale skin should turn pink, while dark skin will be darker. The treatment should occur every two to three hours initially, decreasing to three times a day as healing progresses and the swelling subsides.

Heat should never be used in the acute stage of injury, as it produces vasodilation, increasing blood flow and swelling. Heat may, however, be used after healing has taken place, usually six to twelve days, but only after the bruising turns yellow. Heat is effective at this stage to relax the muscles and improve elasticity before rehabilitative exercise.

COMPRESSION

This has been covered already in the outline of rest and support procedures. Additional pressure can be applied if a layer of cotton wool is applied to the area before bandaging. Do not use non-elasticated bandages on a recent injury, as the strapping needs some stretch to allow for swelling. Check the colour of the skin and nails distal to the injury. Release the bandage if the skin is white and the nails are blue.

ELEVATION

The injured part should be supported in elevation whenever possible. Gravity will then assist the drainage of any fluid exudate away from the area. This will help to reduce the pressure and the pain around the damaged area.

DIAGNOSIS

As previously stated, accurate diagnosis is crucial for maximum recovery. Refer the injured person to a doctor or a hospital casualty department.

Injuries

ACUTE INJURIES

Traumatic injuries happen suddenly due to some external force or internal stress, producing sudden pain, swelling, bruising or wounds.

CHRONIC INJURIES

Repetitive strain injuries or overuse injuries occur slowly, becoming progressively worse over a period of time. Pain is usually of gradual onset but persists over a long period of time.

PREVENTION

It is extremely important to take every precaution to prevent injury occurring: the safety factors are discussed fully in chapter 10.

Important points to remember are:

- Wear appropriate, well-supporting footwear, designed for the activity.
- Select a suitable, safe venue with appropriate facilities and good surfaces.
- Plan appropriate, well-designed exercise schemes showing gradual progression with accurate instruction.
- Maintain good body alignment throughout, and learn correct techniques and correct breathing patterns.
- Perform an adequate and appropriate warm-up and cool-down.
- Allow adequate rest, relaxation and recovery time.
- Ensure that appropriate fitness assessment is performed prior to undertaking sport or exercise and also on return after injury.
- Avoid exercise if there are any contra-indications.

TREATMENT

The more rapidly treatment is administered following injury, the greater the chance of a speedy full recovery. Treatment should start immediately where possible and certainly within 48 hours.

The first priority with traumatic injuries is to assess the situation:

- Check the breathing: watch for chest movement or check the nose and mouth for air flow.
- Check the heartbeat: feel for the radial pulse at the wrist, or the carotid pulse at the throat behind the windpipe.
- Check for broken bones: if for any reason fractures are suspected, do not move the casualty more than is absolutely necessary. This is particularly important if there is damage to the spine. Moving a casualty with damage to his or her spine can result in permanent paralysis.
- Check for bleeding: any profuse bleeding should be stemmed by applying firm, even pressure directly over the area, preferably over a sterile dressing. Avoid direct contact with blood.
- Check for other injuries: look for wounds, cuts, abrasions and signs of joint damage, e.g. pain, ligament sprains, muscle and tendon strain and tears.

The aims of treatment are to:

- prevent further damage;
- reduce the inflammatory response;
- promote healing and reduce pain, swelling and stiffness;
- gradually stretch, mobilise and strengthen the affected tissues;
- maintain the full strength and condition of unaffected body parts;
- return the body to normal function.

PRECAUTIONS

- Do not move a casualty with injuries to the spine.
- Do not move casualties with bone fractures more than is absolutely necessary.
- Apply bandages and strapping firmly but not too tightly, as too much pressure may cut off the circulation.
- Check the limbs beyond the strapping for cold white or blue colouration, which indicates lack of circulation. Loosen the strapping immediately.
- Do not apply heat in any form to the injured area, i.e. do not use heat lamps, hot packs, hot baths, showers, ultrasound, diathermy, hot towels or any liniments.
- Do not massage the injured area.
- Do not exercise through the pain or use EMS (electrical muscle stimulation).

- Do not drink alcohol
  (The previous four actions are to be avoided as they will increase bleeding, exudation and swelling.)
- Seek a medical diagnosis as quickly as possible.
- Apply the RICED principle as soon as possible.
- Ice should be applied for fifteen to thirty minutes every two hours or so initially and then three times a day for the first 48–72 hours. Do not apply ice directly onto the skin: place a tea towel between the skin and the ice, as explained on page 237.

Heat, massage and gentle movement may be used after initial healing has taken place, some six to ten days after injury, but they must not be used if there is any risk of further bleeding.

TYPES OF INJURY

Injuries may occur to any part of the body, and they affect body tissues in different ways.

SKIN AND SUBCUTANEOUS TISSUES

Sharp objects, equipment or apparatus, the playing surface and so on may cause injuries to the skin and underlying tissue. These include cuts, abrasions, infections and contusions.

Protect yourself from contact with blood. Wear rubber surgical gloves if available, or place the hand in a plastic bag. The Hepatitis B and HIV viruses are transmitted through blood contamination.

- Cuts should be thoroughly cleaned and all dirt or debris removed. They should be washed with clean water and/or antiseptic solutions and sterile swabs. Swab from the centre outwards, using a clean swab each time. Then cover with a sterile dressing. Large, gaping cuts more than 2 cm long will require stitching: refer the injured person to a casualty department immediately.
- Abrasions caused by friction or scraping of the skin are usually superficial. Clean them and treat them as cuts.
- Infections of cuts, abrasions or blisters can occur as a result of dirt and micro-organisms penetrating the skin or hair follicles. Infections may result in boils or carbuncles, which may require antibiotics to prevent them spreading to underlying tissues. Refer the casualty to a doctor if infection occurs.
- Contusions (or bruising) of the skin are caused by direct blows and result in bleeding into the tissues. Apply ice directly over the contusion to reduce bleeding and swelling. Do not use heat or massage, as these will increase bleeding.

MUSCLE INJURIES

Injuries to muscles may be strains, partial tears or complete tears.

- Strains will result in micro-tears within some fibres of the muscle. The symptoms, pain and stiffness, are slow in onset and usually mild.

- Partial tears result in the tearing and disruption of some fibres within the muscle. The symptoms are felt immediately, with severe pain and tenderness, especially when attempting to contract the muscle.

- Complete tears result in the tearing of all the muscle fibres, and the two ends of the muscle contract away from each other. There will be severe pain, swelling and complete loss of function. This type of injury requires surgery.

Initially, muscle injuries should be treated with RICE as soon as possible. Any vigorous movements, stretching, heat and massage must be avoided, as complications may result.

TENDON INJURIES

- Tears usually occur at the tendon's weakest point, that is where it joins the muscle at the musculo-tendinous junction. They may be partial tears, when some fibres are torn, or complete tears, when the tendon is severed. Complete tears require surgery; the best results are obtained if surgery is performed immediately, before the two ends shrink and move apart. The pain is immediate, sharp and severe. It feels like a sharp blow to the area and the 'snap' can sometimes be heard.

- Tendinitis (inflammation of a tendon) and tenosynovitis (inflammation of the tendon in its sheath) are very common problems. They are usually caused by repetitive stress or overuse, but can be caused by awkward movements such as landing awkwardly or mis-hitting a ball. The pain is niggling and comes on gradually. It is worse when the tendon is moved and may progress until movements are impossible. Because the blood supply to tendons is poor they can take a very long time to heal: up to twelve weeks or even longer.

LIGAMENT INJURIES

Ligaments attach bone to bone. They support and stabilise joints. Ligaments are damaged when joints are forced into abnormal positions.

- Sprains occur when a few fibres are torn, producing pain and swelling. These heal quickly, with little disruption of joint movement.

- Partial tears occur when a number of fibres are torn due to greater stress. These produce severe pain and swelling and the joint will be unstable.
- Complete tears are very severe, producing extreme pain and swelling, and the joint will be quite unstable and may dislocate. Torn ligaments may heal well without surgery, but others will require suturing.

INJURIES TO MENISCI

The menisci are discs of cartilage found in certain joints: for example, in the knee the medial and lateral menisci lie on the upper surface of the condyles of the tibia. They may tear due to excessive forces during rotation or extreme flexion, causing acute pain and swelling. The knee may lock if a part of the disc becomes dislodged and interferes with the function of the knee. Surgery may be required to remove part of the cartilage, but some tears heal without surgery.

INJURIES TO BURSAE

Bursae are sacs of fluid that reduce friction between the moving parts of a joint. They lie between tendons and bones and allow smooth movement of the tendon over the bone. They can become inflamed, usually due to overuse or repetitive trauma.

Inflammation of a bursa is known as bursitis; it produces pain and swelling in the area of the bursa and radiating pain around it. It may heal with rest or may require a cortisone injection to help it settle. Very occasionally, surgery is required for a persistently painful bursa.

FRACTURES

A fracture is a break in a bone. Fractures may be simple or compound. A simple fracture is a clean break in the bone. A compound fracture involves more complex breaks of the bone and perforation of the skin.

Bones fracture due to excessive force applied to the bone. Stress or fatigue fractures occur as a result of overuse, when repetitive muscle contraction pulls on the bone, causing repeated minor stress and damage which does not have time to heal.

Fractures require immobilisation in order to reduce the displacement and prevent movement, allowing time for the fracture to heal. Fractures of the upper limb usually heal in six to eight weeks, providing there are no complications such as inadequate blood supply. However, lower limb fractures take twelve to fourteen weeks. Fractures heal more quickly in children than adults.

Common injuries

While it is not possible to cover all injuries and their treatment in this book, examples of common injuries are included. Students who require more detailed knowledge must refer to specific medical books.

The following are examples of common injuries, including first aid guidelines.

Table 15.1 *Foot and ankle joint injuries*

Injury	*Cause*	*Action*
Stress fractures	caused by repetitive stress to the small bones of the foot due to long-distance running, marching, etc. Pain over the site of the fracture	RICED. Stop activity until healing is complete. Wear shoes with adequate firm soles
Plantar fascitis: the fascia on the sole of the foot becomes inflamed	caused by change of footwear, excessive or different movements performed by the foot. Pain just in front of or over the heel	RICED. A sponge shock absorber under the heel may help
Spring ligament strain	caused by over-stretching of the spring ligament in the sole of the foot through excessive walking, running, jumping, etc. Pain is felt in the sole	RICED. Wear well-supporting shoes; arch support may help
Bursitis: inflammation of the bursa between the Achilles tendon and calcaneus	caused by rubbing of ill-fitting shoes. Pain and tenderness are felt at the back of the heel	RICED. Change footwear, making sure the heel tab is low and not rubbing
Achilles tendon, partial rupture	caused by sudden stretching when muscles are cold or tired. Sudden pain is felt over the tendon or in the calf	RICED. May take six weeks to heal. Use massage and gentle stretch to recover normal function
Achilles tendon, complete rupture	again caused by severe stretching of the tendon when muscles are tired or cold. A sudden severe pain is felt in the calf, as if the person has been kicked. Walking is very difficult. Standing on tip-toe on one leg is impossible	RICED. Seek medical advice immediately, as surgery is nearly always necessary to suture the ends of the tendon together

Tendinitis and tenosynovitis	pain and tenderness are felt along the tendon. Stiffness develops and crepitus (a grating sound) may be heard as the tendon moves in the sheath. Caused by excessive use of the tendon or rubbing of ill-fitting shoes. May occur to any of the tendons around the foot or wrist	RICED. May take six weeks or more to settle. Avoid all activities that produce pain and crepitus
Tendon strain	may occur to any of the long tendons around the foot and ankle. Pain is felt along the tendon	RICED. Wear well-fitting shoes with good support. Ensure good technique and adequate warm-up
Sprained ankle: a very common injury that may affect the medial ligament of the ankle but more usually affects the outer lateral ligament, as there is a greater range of movement when turning foot inwards (inversion)	occurs when the foot 'turns over'. Pain and tenderness are felt over the site of the injury. There may be bruising and swelling. Depending on the extent of the injury. The ligaments may rupture and the malleoli may fracture	RICED. It is important to obtain an accurate diagnosis quickly, as the ankle may need strapping or a plaster cast. Ice and elevation must start immediately and continue for 48 hours. Crutches may be needed to take the weight off the ankle
Unstable ankle	following ankle sprains the ankle may 'give way' at times because full function has not returned	an accurate diagnosis is essential. Strapping may be necessary. Exercises will strengthen the surrounding muscles
Fractures	severe trauma can cause a fracture of either the fibular or the tibial malleolus, or both may fracture. There will be pain, swelling and bruising. All movement of the ankle will hurt and it may be impossible to walk	RICED. Immediate diagnosis is required. A strapping or plaster cast is applied to prevent further damage. Surgery is sometimes needed to pin the bones
Footballer's ankle	pain and stiffness of the ankle as a result of repeated trauma and kicks to the ankle. The ligaments are damaged and new bone spurs may develop	RICED. Use strapping and shin pads to protect against further injury
Blisters	caused by rubbing of ill-fitting shoes or by excessive activity	allow the blister time to heal. Keep the area clean to avoid infection. Check and change shoes if necessary

Table 15.2 *Lower leg injuries*

Injury	Cause	Action
Muscle pain and strain	this may happen to any of the muscles of the lower leg: anterior pain or strain of the muscles in front of the shin that dorsi-flex the foot; posterior pain or strain of the muscles of the calf that plantar flex the foot; lateral pain or strain of the lateral muscles that pull the foot outwards (eversion); medial pain or strain of the muscles that pull the foot inwards (inversion)	RICE. Reduce activities and change training schedules. Analyse and develop a correct technique
Shin splints: pain over the front and outer side of the shin bone. The nagging ache comes on slowly, but may develop into a deep pain and extreme tenderness	the constant and repetitive pulling of the muscles on the tibia produces microscopic tearing of the muscle attachments. It is caused by many factors, including inadequate warm-up, lack of flexibility, poor technique, overuse, fatigue, or running on hard surfaces	RICED. Return to training very gradually, ensure adequate warm-up and flexibility, work on spring floors and proper tracks. Wear well-supporting cushion-soled shoes
Stress fractures	similar to shin splint pain and caused by repetitive stress to the tibia as above. The bone cracks and is not given the chance to heal	RICED. Rest for six weeks or more; may need immobilisation in plaster. Return to training very gradually as above
Simple and compound fractures of the tibia or fibula	caused by direct trauma to the lower leg. They are common in soccer and rugby players	RICED. Seek diagnosis immediately. The leg will need a plaster cast and sometimes surgery. Recovery can take three months or more
Pain over the tibial tubercle: the point of attachment of the quadriceps tendon	caused by an excessive, sudden pull of the tendon, e.g. during deep squats or weight lifting. It may also be caused by long-distance running. Pain is felt over the tubercle and also within the muscle when it contracts. The tendon may tear or may pull away a flake of bone	RICED. Allow sufficient time to heal and avoid stress on the tendon

KNEE INJURIES

The knee has a complicated hinge structure and is vulnerable to numerous injuries, both internal and external. Sudden severe swelling indicates a severe type of injury, such as a complete rupture of the ligaments or cartilage or a fracture. Slow swelling over twelve hours or more indicates less severe trauma, such as a torn cartilage, sprained ligaments or damage of the synovial membrane.

Table 15.3 *Knee injuries*

Injury	*Cause*	*Action*
Medial ligament sprains and tears:	caused by forcing the lower leg outwards. Fibres may stretch, tear or completely rupture. Pain is felt on the inner side of the knee: it may be mild or severe. Frequently happens when skiing, during football tackles or through slipping when running. More common than lateral ligament injuries	RICED. Immediate diagnosis is necessary. It may need splinting, a plaster cast or surgery depending on the severity of the injury
Lateral ligament sprains and tears	as above, except that they occur when the lower leg is forced inwards; the pain is felt on the lateral aspect of the knee	RICED. Usually less severe than medial ligament injury
Dislocation of the patella: the kneecap is forced sideways out of alignment	caused by a sudden twist on a straight knee or a blow to the knee. It frequently occurs in children. A sharp pain is felt, the knee gives way, and this is followed by swelling. May recur	RICED. Do not force back into place. Immediate diagnosis is needed, as it may require reduction (putting back) and splinting. Build up the quadriceps muscle to prevent recurrence
Cartilage injury: a very common injury of one or both of the menisci (the semilunar cartilages of the knee)	usually results from twisting the body on a bent weight-bearing knee or sitting back on the haunches with the feet splayed outwards and rocking backwards. Pain is felt and the knee may give way or lock. Gradual swelling will follow. It may be impossible to straighten the knee	RICED. Seek immediate diagnosis. The tear may be severe and require keyhole surgery to remove part of the cartilage, or it may heal and recover without surgery. Build up the quadriceps before resuming normal activity
Cartilage ligament injury	caused by incorrect technique when running. The ligament which attaches the cartilage to the edge of the joint may be pinched between the tibia and femur and may become inflamed	RICED. Reduce activity, reassess and modify technique
Cruciate ligament rupture	the anterior and posterior cruciate ligaments play a crucial role in the stability of the knee preventing forward	RICED. Seek immediate medical advice, as surgery may be required to suture the ligaments. Strengthen all the muscles

and backward movement of the knee. They will tear if the leg is severely twisted or forced backwards when weight-bearing. One or both cruciates may tear, depending on the force of the injury. Other ligaments may tear at the same time. Severe injury will cause pain and swelling and the knee will feel floppy

around the joint before resuming activities. After surgery and rehabilitation it is wise to avoid contact sports

Muscle strains and tears: these can happen to any of the thigh muscles: to the quadriceps on the front of the thigh, the hamstrings on the back of the thigh or the adductors on the medial aspect

Muscle strains may occur due to over-use, when muscles become tired and less efficient. Pain develops gradually, with tenderness and stiffness but without swelling or bruising
Muscle tears may be partial tears or complete ruptures, depending on the severity of the blow or injury. Pain is immediate and searing with varying degrees of swelling and bruising

RICED. Avoid the activity causing the problem and begin rehabilitation. Ensure adequate warm-up, and stretch and introduce activity gradually. Muscle tears and ruptures must be referred to a doctor as they may require surgery

Direct blow injuries

may be caused by a kick or a blow from apparatus, etc. They vary in severity depending on the strength of the blow. If the muscle is contracted at the time of the blow the fibres may tear. Pain is immediate, stiffness and swelling follow. There may be severe internal bleeding, forming a haematoma. If this heals with some formation of bone there will be some functional loss

RICED. Seek immediate diagnosis. The success of the recovery depends on early correct treatment

Fractures

considerable force is required to fracture the large femur, but it may occur as a result of violent injury. The surrounding muscles and skin may also be damaged

immobilise and seek medical advice immediately

PELVIC INJURIES

The pelvis is a very stable structure, formed by the two innominate bones and the sacrum. Problems may be felt around the hip joint, in the groin, over the pubic symphysis or over the coccyx.

Table 15.4 *Pelvic injuries*

Injury	Cause	Action
Footballer's groin: inflammation at the symphysis pubis	the ligament may be strained due to movement sideways, i.e. side-stepping, hurdling or slipping. Pain is felt over the pubic bone	rest, avoiding the activity that caused the problem
Adductor strain	similar to the above and caused in the same way, but pain is deep in the groin and upon adduction	RICE. Then gradual stretching of the adductors
Pain in the hip joint	may be due to a number of conditions, such as osteo-arthritis, bursitis, etc.	refer to a doctor for accurate diagnosis
Coccydynia: pain at the very base of the spine	usually due to a fall on the tail. May be caused by persistent trauma such as practising excessive sit-ups on a hard floor	apply ice immediately. May take a long time to heal. Seek medical advice if pain persists

SHOULDER AND ARM INJURIES

The shoulder joint is a loose-fitting ball and socket joint that allows a wide range of movement. It has a loose capsule and numerous tendons which support the joint.

Table 15.5 *Shoulder and arm injuries*

Injury	Cause	Action
Muscle strains, tears and ruptures	the muscles and tendons around the joint may be strained gradually through overuse or strained suddenly through direct injury. Overuse injuries occur in swimming, rowing, tennis, shot putting, bowling or weight lifting. Traumatic injuries occur in gymnastics, riding, pole vaulting, parachuting, etc. The muscles may be strained, partially torn or completely ruptured and the pain and stiffness will vary accordingly	RID. Rest from the activity that caused the injury is essential until healing has taken place. A sling may be necessary. Build up strength gradually before resuming the activity

Dislocated shoulder: the capsule of the shoulder is loose and the head of the humerus can be wrenched out of the shallow glenoid cavity	caused by forcing the arm outwards away from the body. Extreme pain is felt immediately and movement is limited or impossible. A common injury in rugby and judo	seek medical advice immediately as the joint needs to be reduced (put back). This must be done by a doctor who knows what to do, as further complications can develop. A sling should be worn for three to six weeks, then build up the strength gradually
Fractures	any of the shoulder girdle or arm bones may fracture. Common fractures are those of the clavicle, the surgical neck of the humerus, the distal end of the radius, the scaphoid and the ribs. Immediate pain is felt following the trauma, with swelling and bruising depending on the type of fracture	refer immediately to a doctor or hospital casualty department
Frozen shoulder: inflammation of the lining of the shoulder joint	may be caused by repetitive trauma. Pain and stiffness are felt in the shoulder and movement becomes increasingly limited	RID. Seek medical advice as other therapies may be effective. Can be very slow to recover: from two months to two years
Bursitis: inflammation of the various bursae around the shoulder joint, e.g. the sub-deltoid or subacromial, or the olecranon bursa at the elbow	will produce pain and stiffness around the joint	RID. Seek medical advice as other therapies may be effective. An injection may be needed
Tennis elbow: strain of the common extensor tendon over the lateral epicondyle of the humerus	caused by wrenching, repetitive stress or incorrect technique. Pain is felt over the lateral epicondyle because the tendon becomes inflamed at its insertion. It hurts to extend the wrist with a bent elbow or when straightening the elbow. Affects tennis players, badminton players and throwers. May occur following any repetitive stress such as lifting, chopping wood or using a screwdriver	RI: rest from the activity, and ice. It may need an injection of cortisone or an operation to release the tendon if the condition persists
Golfer's elbow: the same as tennis elbow, but this is an inflammation of the flexor tendon insertion on the medial epicondyle of the humerus	caused by overuse and stretching of the muscles, a common problem for golfers or javelin throwers. Pain is felt over the medial epicondyle	RI: rest from activity, and ice. It may need an anti-inflammatory injection if the condition persists
Tendinitis and tenosynovitis: inflammation of the tendons within their sheaths where they pass over the wrist	pain and tenderness is felt along the tendon and crepetis may be heard. Movement is painful. Caused by over-use, repetitive movements and faulty technique	RID. Avoid unnecessary movements. A splint may be necessary to provide support

Sprained wrist	caused by excessive stress and movement of the wrist. The ligaments are sprained, with pain and swelling	RICED. Strapping or splinting may be necessary. May require a plaster cast. Resume movements very slowly

Many other injuries can affect the hand and wrist. Always seek medical advice, as function may be impaired through lack of correct treatment.

CHEST INJURIES

Injury to the chest may result in fractures of one or more ribs. It is unusual to suffer muscle strain unless it accompanies rib fractures.

Possible injuries are:

- Fractures of the ribs
- Stress fractures of the ribs
- Fractures of the sternum.

Causes of the fractures may be as follows:

- Rib or sternum fractures are caused by severe stress, such as falling awkwardly and hitting the chest on some hard object or being hit by a cricket or tennis ball, etc.
- Stress fractures are caused by repetitive stress and excessive use of the chest muscles, as in tennis or shot putting.

Seek medical advice for an accurate diagnosis, but little is done for fractured ribs as they are well held by the intercostal muscles.

Fractured ribs may sometimes puncture the underlying lung, producing intense pain, breathlessness and pallid skin. In this case the casualty should be taken to hospital immediately.

INJURIES TO THE VERTEBRAL COLUMN

Any area of the vertebral column is susceptible to injury, but most injuries are sustained in the lumbar and cervical regions.

The injuries that may be sustained are:

- Fractures of the vertebrae
- Sprains and tears of the supporting ligaments
- Strains and tears of the supporting muscles
- Damage or prolapse of the inter-vertebral discs.

Causes of injury may be as follows:

- Fractures are usually caused by severe stress, as in falling from a height, motor accidents, parachute jumping, hard rugby tackles, etc.

- The tearing of ligaments and muscle fibres is caused by sudden overload.
- Strains and sprains are caused by repetitive stress overload, and by awkward or inappropriate movements.
- Disc damage is caused by suddenly increased compression forces, as occur when lifting heavy weights, when lifting at an awkward angle, or because of poor postural care during exercise and movement. Trunk forward flexion exercises can damage the lumbar spine and the head circling exercise can damage the cervical spine (see chapter 11).

All severe back injuries must be approached with great care. **Do not** move the casualty unless it is essential for resuscitation to save life. The spinal column protects the spinal cord, which runs through the vertebral foramen. Any fracture of the vertebrae can increase pressure on the cord, partially damage it or sever it completely. These injuries may result in partial or total paralysis from that level downwards. Moving the casualty will increase the risk of cord damage. Seek medical help immediately. All back injuries must be medically referred, including gradual back pain that becomes progressively worse.

Practice Tasks

Explain how and why you would teach a client to breathe correctly (refer to pages 5, 39–40):

Explain how you would instruct a client to get down on to the floor and come up again (refer to page 230):

Devise a record card that you would use during the initial consultation and assessment of each client, prior to their exercise classes (refer to chapter 10):

Study a variety of exercise videos, exercise books and magazine articles and complete the following tasks.

List any exercises that you would consider unsafe:

Devise your own set of warm-up exercises:

Devise a set of aerobic exercises:

Devise a set of cool-down exercises:

References and further reading

Alter, Michael J. (1988), *Science of Sketching*, Human Kinetics Books.
An excellent book for anyone requiring any information on flexibility work.

American Council on Exercise (1991), *Aerobic Dance-Exercise Instructors Manual.*
A useful source of detailed information for anyone leading aerobic classes.

Beashel, Paul, and Taylor, John (1988) *Sport Examined*, Macmillan Education.

Cross, Gibbs and Gray (1991), *The Sporting Body*, Sydney: McGraw Hill Book Co.

Curzon, L.B. (1976), *Teaching in Further Education*, London: Cassell.

Daniels, Lucille, and Worthington, Catherine (1977), *Therapeutic Exercise*, WB Saunders Co.
Comprehensive information on correction and maintenance of posture and body alignment.

Davies, Kimmel and Anly (1988), *Physical Education Theory & Practice*, Macmillan Company (Australia).
Covers the detail of exercise theory. Interesting additional reading.

Grisogono, Vivian (1984), *Sports Injuries*, London: John Murray.
A good self-help guide on the avoidance and treatment of sports injuries.

Hazeldine, R. (1993), *Fitness for Sport*, The Crowood Press.
Excellent, clearly explained information for individuals training for or teaching the theory of fitness. Good examples of exercise programmes, circuits, etc., for achieving set goals.

Kennedy, Legel and Sagamore (1992), *Anatomy of an Exercise Class*, Human Kinetics Books. Gives detailed information on the degrees of movement possible at body joints. Excellent information on analysis of exercises.

Luby, Sue, and St Onge, Richard A. (1986), *Body Sense*, Faber & Faber Inc.
A well-illustrated book clearly showing the hazards of poor postural alignment. Covers the fundamentals of breathing, posture and alignment, stretching techniques and other useful topics.

Sharkey, B.J. (1990), *Physiology of Fitness*, Human Kinetics Books. Gives detailed information on the physiological aspects of exercise.

Smith, B. (1993), *Advanced Fitness Teachers Manual*, Ludoe Publications (Loughborough University).
Gives specific information on training for the components of fitness.

St George, Francine (1990), *The Muscle Fitness Book*, The Crowood Press.
Good guidelines on safe, effective exercise for specific sporting activities.

Time-Life Books (1990), *Cross Training – Ultimate Fitness*.
Interesting reading for those interested in the concept of cross training. A good chapter on 'Eating for Performance' gives recipes for suitable foods.

Index